THE MANAGEMENT OF PERSONS
WITH SPINAL CORD INJURY

The Management of Persons with Spinal Cord Injury

Mark N. Ozer, M.D.

*Associate Professor of Neurology
Medical College of Virginia
and
Assistant Chief, SCI Service
H. H. McGuire VA Medical Center
Richmond, Virginia*

DEMOS PUBLICATIONS
New York

Demos Publications, 156 Fifth Avenue, New York, New York 10010

©1988 by Demos Publications, Inc. All rights reserved. This book is protected by copyright. No part of it may be reproduced, stored in a retrieval system, or transmitted in any form or by any means, electronic, mechanical, photocopying, recording, or otherwise, without the prior written permission of the publisher.

Made in the United States of America

Great care has been taken to maintain the accuracy of the information contained in this volume. However, Dr. Mark N. Ozer and Demos Publications cannot be held responsible for errors or for any consequences arising from the use of the information contained herein.

ISBN: 0-939957-10-8

LC: 88-070004

Preface

The treatment of the person with spinal cord injury (SCI) affords health professionals the extraordinary opportunity to view the long-term physical effects of neurological injury and to contribute over an extended period of time to the total care of a person who must learn to live his life with a disability. In describing the features of SCI and summarizing the multi-faceted issues relevant to the care of the spinal-cord-injured person during all phases of recovery, this book should prove useful to those in a wide variety of disciplines—physicians working with patients with SCI, particularly residents in neurology and rehabilitation medicine, physical therapists, occupational therapists, nurses, and others seeking a basic introduction to this field.

This book sets out to provide a background set of principles and to review state-of-the art techniques of diagnosis and treatment. It emphasizes the growing trend of encouraging the individual with SCI to participate in defining the nature of his disabilities and in solving problems related to them. Its contents closely follow the evolution of the newly spinal-cord-injured person; an introductory chapter outlining basic principles of SCI management is followed by chapters devoted to each major phase of the post-injury period, with special emphasis on rehabilitation. For each of these phases, the goals are defined, the problems encountered are delineated, and treatment solutions are offered. It will become readily apparent that, whereas minimizing *impairment* is the goal initially, minimizing *disability* and maximizing *health* and fostering integration into the community become paramount in the goal-setting process later on.

It will also be demonstrated how the character of interaction between the person with SCI and the health care system changes as the person begins to contribute to his own care and to participate in planning for his future. The successful management of chronic neurological impairment largely depends on the injured person developing pragmatic problem-solving approaches appropriate for his own personal rehabilitation and continuing care with the help of the health professional. A specific method for achieving this collaboration is discussed in detail in the final chapter on participatory planning.

The idea for this book arose out of my need, upon return to clinical work, to learn about the care of persons with SCI in the context of my long-standing interest in developing new models of health care for persons with disabilities. I would like to thank Dr. Diana M. Schneider and Dr. Labe Scheinberg, whose advice during the genesis of this project was invaluable, and Dr. Nelson Richards and Dr. Norman Bass for their encouragement and helpful suggestions. I am particularly grateful to the patients of the SCI Service at the McGuire VA Medical Center in Richmond, to my colleagues on the professional staff, to Anne Meader of the secretarial staff, and to the chief of service, Dr. Robert W. Hussey, to whom this book is dedicated.

Contents

1. Principles of Spinal Cord Injury Management 1
   The Nature of the Problem 1
     The spinal cord
     The person with SCI
     The environment
     The natural history of SCI
   The Character of the Solution 7

2. Acute Care 13
   The Nature of the Injury 13
     Neurological aspects
     Orthopedic aspects
   Treatment Approaches 22

3. Rehabilitation 29
   Impairments and Disabilities 30
     Sensation
     Motor function
     Micturition
     Defecation
     Sexual function
     Autonomic function
   Minimizing Disabilities 56
     Bladder retraining
     Bowel retraining
     Sexual reintegration
     Skin management
     Mobility retraining
     Activities of daily living
     Breathing
   The Goals of Rehabilitation 78

4. Continuing Care	87
Problems in Continuing Care	*88*
Post-traumatic syringomyelia	
The management of spasticity	
The management of chronic pain	
5. Participatory Planning	107
The Problem	*107*
The Goal	*108*
The Method	*109*
Index	115

CHAPTER *1*

Principles of Spinal Cord Injury Management

THE NATURE OF THE PROBLEM

The incidence of persons with spinal cord injury (SCI) requiring care has been variously calculated, with the most acceptable figure being in the range of 8,000–9,000 new cases per year in the United States (1). With the increase of longevity post-injury, the prevalence of this problem is generally calculated to be in the range of 200,000 persons. Medical costs associated with the care of this population during their initial hospitalization and subsequent follow-up care have been calculated to be over $1.5 billion (1981 dollars). This figure does not include societal costs, which are less easily determined but may be far greater, such as attendant care, vocational rehabilitation, income maintenance, and loss of income, as well as environmental modifications to increase physical accessibility.

Since World War II, SCI centers have been established throughout the world to provide comprehensive care designed to prevent the early mortality and high morbidity previously associated with this problem. Such multidisciplinary centers also provide a model of continuity of care, including ongoing follow-up services to deal with both medical and surgical complications and their prevention. This book deals with the health care of persons with SCI as developed in such centers (2,3).

The kinds of problems the person with SCI brings to the health care professional are the result of both the extent of the injury and the unique characteristics of each individual.

The spinal cord

The anatomy of the spinal cord—its osseus/ligamentous supports, its vascular supply, and its internal organization—greatly but not entirely determines the effects of an injury. In general, approximately half of those who are alive on arrival at a hospital are paraplegic, a majority of whom have a loss of sensory or motor function below the level of the lesion ("complete"). Of the other half, with involvement at the level of the cervical cord, a somewhat higher percentage experience preservation of some sensation of motor function below the level of the lesion ("incomplete") (1). The number of incomplete cervical injuries has been increasing recently; this has been attributed to improvements in emergency procedures to protect the spinal cord from further damage.

The spinal cord extends from below the foramen magnum to the second lumbar vertebra (Fig. 1-1). The L4-L5 segmental level of the cord is situated at the T11-T12 vertebral interspace; S2 cord level at the T12-L1 interspace; and S4 level approximately at the L1 interspace. Injuries are more common in an area where a highly mobile vertebral segment joins a less mobile segment, such as the lower cervical region and the thoracolumbar junction.

The spinal cord occupies approximately one-third of the area enclosed by the arch of the atlas. In the remainder of the cervical area, 50% of the spinal canal is occupied by the cord. There is special hazard to the effects of compression at C5, where the cord is at its greatest width because of the cervical enlargement. The free play available within the subarachnoid space is particularly diminished in extension of the neck. Buckling of the ligamentum flavum posteriorly and bulging of the discs and spondyltic ridges anteriorly are more evident in the elderly, with even greater likelihood of compromise of the cord in extension (4).

The high incidence of complete lesions with injuries in the thoracic cord is attributed to the relative narrowness of the thoracic canal between T1-T10 (5). The thickest part of the cord is located between T10 and T12, with a resultant reduction in free play at those segments. The character of the blood supply to the thoracic region also leads to particular problems in perfusion in the area of T5 and L1. Within the cord itself, the central grey matter and the ventral portion of the posterior columns represent weak points in the circulation. Relative sparing of the sacral motor and sensory function with ischemia in the central portion of the cord reflects the lamination of the tracts, with the caudal portion most lateral in both the corticospinal and spinothalamic tracts (see Fig. 1-2). The relative vulnerability of the anterior portion of the cord is attributed to the unpaired nature of the anterior spinal artery, whereas the pair of posterior spinal arteries tends to protect that portion from the effects of damage (6) (see Fig. 1-3). In the lumbar region, the canal is considerably larger. Since the cord ends at the L1-L2 vertebral level and the ca-

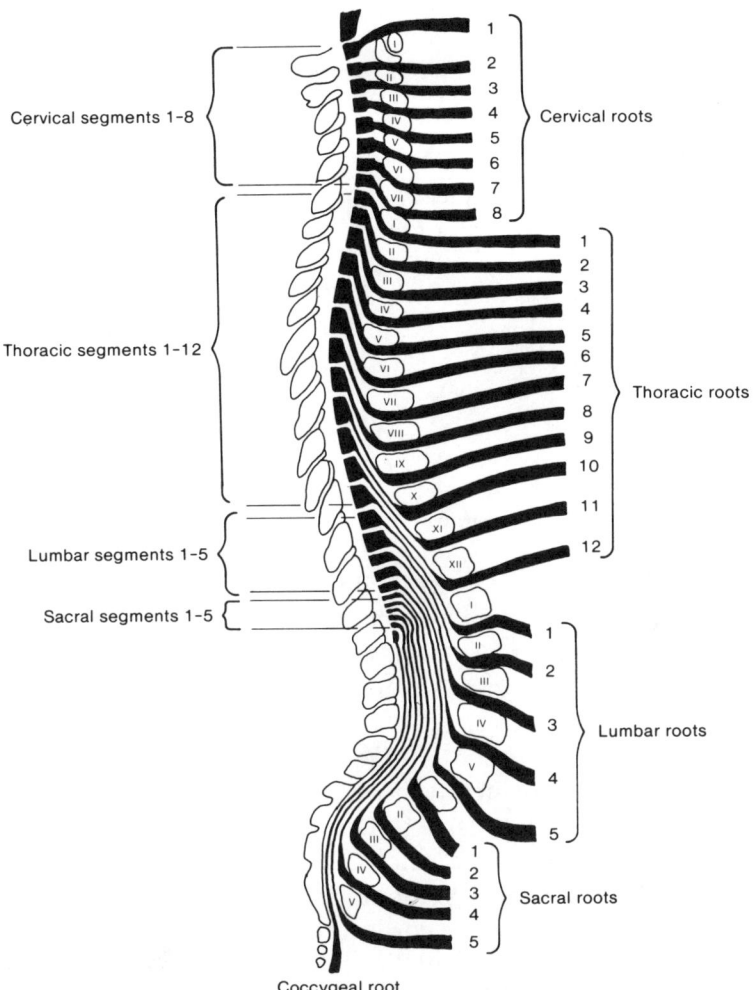

FIG. 1-1. The structure of the spinal cord showing the correlation between the spinal cord segments and nerve roots. (Adapted by permission from ref. 6, 14th ed.)

nal contains only the roots of the cauda equina, a large amount of free space is available. Thus, a significant displacement of the vertebral bodies is required to produce any neurological impairment at this segment (7).

Ten-year survival, although much improved from that in the past, is still highly affected by the presence of SCI and the degree of injury. The likelihood of death is increased approximately six- to sevenfold in those with paraplegia as compared to normal controls, with little difference

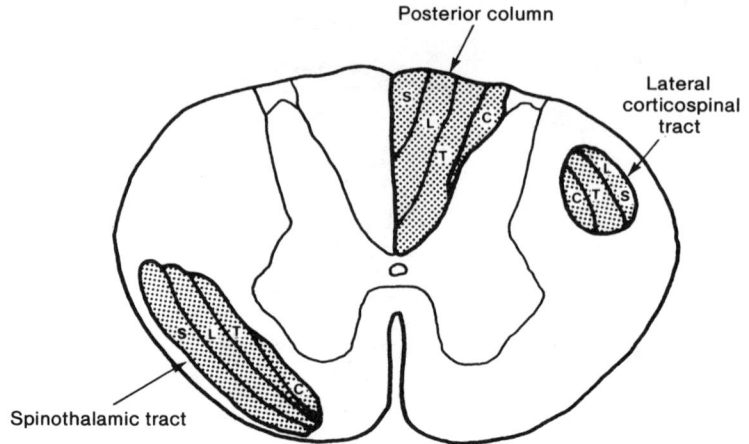

FIG. 1-2. Lamination of the spinal cord tracts. C, cervical; L, lumbar; S, sacral; T, thoracic. (Adapted from ref. 6.)

between those with complete or incomplete lesions. The likelihood of deaths within 10 years in those with quadriplegia whose lesions were incomplete was increased 10-fold, whereas those whose lesions were complete had a 20-fold increase compared to the expected mortality for their age group (8).

The effects of SCI frequently extend beyond the neurological and spinal skeletal systems to include injuries to other body systems, such as other bones as well as soft tissues. During the acute phase, there are a large number of associated cardiothoracic and abdominal injuries in those with thoracic cord involvement. This results from the high energy impact required to disrupt the cord in this region protected by the rib cage. Major causes of morbidity throughout the life of the person with SCI are problems with the urinary tract, skin, and gastrointestinal systems. See Hussey (9) for a description of the application of a standardized problem list to SCI.

In clarifying the interaction of the person and the injury, it is useful to use the well-established distinction made between "impairment" and "disability" (10). "Impairment" describes the loss of sensation or coordination of motor actions or loss of autonomic control of urination, bowel evacuation, and sexual function that may occur with damage to the spinal cord or roots, while "disability" refers to the functional consequences of such impairments: the activities in the life of the person that have been affected. For example, the impairment in motor coordination called "paraplegia" generally leads to a disability in mobility. The loss of sensation of fullness in the bladder may lead to inability to

PRINCIPLES OF SPINAL CORD INJURY MANAGEMENT

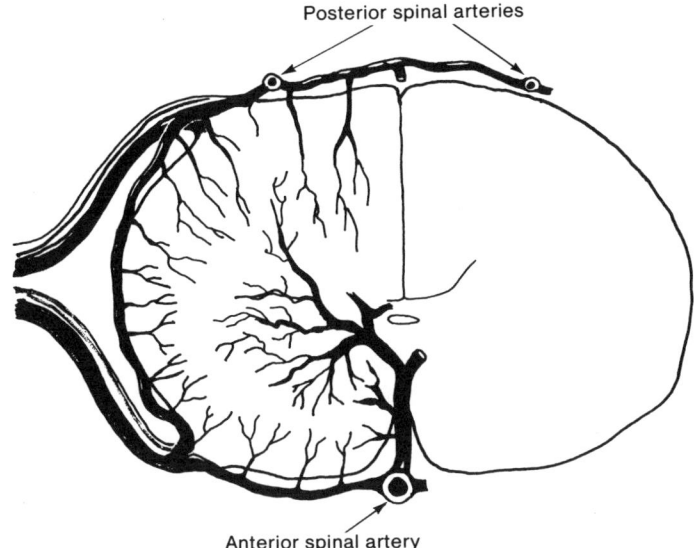

FIG. 1-3. The arterial blood supply of the spinal cord showing the single anterior spinal artery and paired posterior spinal arteries. (Adapted by permission from ref. 6, 14th ed.)

empty the urinary bladder at the appropriate time and place. *It is important to recognize that it is frequently possible to effect change in these disabilities even if the impairments continue to exist.*

The person with SCI

The functional consequences of impairments (disabilities) will vary from person to person. In the case of most new injuries, the person is most frequently a male (4:1), injured in a motor vehicle, in a diving or other sports-related accident, or by a knife or gunshot. Although the greatest frequency is in young males, motor vehicle accidents continue to be the leading cause of SCI in all age groups, with a relative increase in injuries due to falls in older persons. There is a greater difference between observed and expected survival with advancing age, suggesting that the effects of SCI become more life-threatening. In the study by Young et al. (1), the median age, however, was 25, with the mode at age 19 and almost half not yet high school graduates. Because of both their relative youthfulness and educational level, many persons with SCI may be expected to be more likely to act than to be reflective, and not be as likely to be aware of the consequences of their acts (11). Thus, a person who has not perhaps developed a sense of control over many aspects of his life is confronted, for example, with an impairment of voluntary musculature which signifies a loss of some of the controls he has achieved. Especially devastating might be the loss of control over physical action for a person who may have particularly prided himself on his physical prowess.

The environment

Functional problems or disabilities vary not only with the person in whom the impairments exist but also in the interaction of that person with the environment in which he acts. The term "handicap" has been used to describe the contribution to the disabilities by the limitations in the environment (10). For example, a person with paraplegia has disabilities in mobility in an environment in which doorways are too narrow for wheelchairs and stairs block entrances. One major part of the environment in which the person with SCI must interact is the setting in which rehabilitation and health care are carried out. It is important for those acting within the health care system to recognize themselves as having an effect on persons with SCI (12). A major goal of this volume is to enable such individuals to not inadvertently handicap the patient's ability to re-establish control over his life activities, and thus to alleviate the effects of SCI.

It is therefore necessary at the outset to view the problems of SCI as a result of the interaction of these multiple factors: the degree and type of impairment; the person with the impairment; and the physical and social environment, of which the health care system forms a significant part.

The natural history of SCI

The natural history of SCI is of a usually abrupt nonprogressive disruption of the spinal cord. The prototype etiology is an actual physical disruption of the cord or its vascular supply by trauma. Although a similar clinical picture can occur with the other etiologies such as primary vascular disease or inflammatory disease, this volume deals primarily with the pattern of classic SCI due to trauma. Once the initial disruption in function has occurred, there will not ordinarily be any further progression.

The life cycle of the person with SCI involves three unequal phases during which the nature of the problem changes. The first portion of life post-injury—lasting hours to days—is that of acute care concerned with maintaining life and minimizing damage to the spinal cord. The goal is to prevent further "impairment" and the loss of activities controlled by the cord through appropriate medical and surgical interventions. The completion of this phase is generally marked by the achievement of medical stabilization and the carrying out of definitive surgical stabilization when indicated. A high level of professional involvement is required in this acute care stage. The risk of dying due to medical proglems is greatest during this early period post-injury (4.4%) (13).

The second stage—lasting weeks to months—is concerned with restoration. The goal of the rehabilitation phase is to minimize disability despite the continuation of impairment. Alternative means of meeting daily needs are frequently necessary in order to lessen the disabilities. The person must become aware both of the possibility of alternative means and of what specific techniques may be appropriate for his or her specific impairments. Although the person generally remains in a hospital during this period, the intensity of professional involvement is somewhat less and follows a model compatible with an educational setting rather than a strictly medical one. The professionals involved are more varied and form the traditional rehabilitation team, requiring considerable coordination in their interaction with the patient.

The third stage—lasting years—is concerned with continuing care. The goal is to continue to minimize disability by maximizing "health," the ability to function on one's own in the community outside of the hospital, largely independent of ongoing interaction with the health care system. The attainment of this goal requires those with SCI to put into daily practice health care skills learned during their hospitalization post-injury. While there has been a major reduction in deaths due to diseases of the genitourinary system (14), urinary tract infections remain the most common cause for morbidity in the long term, followed by (1) skin problems and spasms as the next most frequent causes for morbidity and hospitalization.

THE CHARACTER OF THE SOLUTION

The goal of this volume is to provide all those concerned with the management of the spinal cord injured person with the information and the procedures that will enable them to deal with all three phases discussed above, and to provide a continuity of care often missing, to the great disadvantage of the person with SCI. In accordance with the goal of minimizing handicaps created within the health care system, it is particularly necessary to recognize the changes in the role of the physician and other health professionals from that seen in the acute care system. In addition to the already well-established principles of comprehensive care and continuity of care must be added the principle of the provision of care in collaboration with the person with SCI. The ultimate test of the physician's skill is the ability of the person with SCI to manage his or her life, with particular emphasis on the management of health care. The role of the physician must evolve into that of a consultant, with the primary responsibility for health belonging to the person with SCI. This approach is discussed in detail in Chapter 5.

Particularly indicative of this evolution of roles is the method by which information is collected about the nature of the problem and the use to which such information is put at these various stages.

During the acute care stage, the goal of examination is to determine the degree and type of impairment and its possible remediation. The primary concern is the existence of paraplegia and sensory losses of various sorts, as determined by the classic neurological examination. Because the focus is on signs found during the physical examination, the patient may be a relatively passive participant in this process.

During rehabilitation, the goal of information collection becomes the determination of disability and its remediation. The neurological examination is no longer the most appropriate means for such a determination. Identifying the existence and the character of a disability requires a major contribution by the patient. Discussion no longer centers on physical changes, such as those involving certain organs or systems of the body, but rather on the adjustment in activities or functions the patient has to effect because of the injury.

Any particular impairment, such as weakness of the lower extremities, may have substantially different consequences for different people. One person after an accident viewed the effects of the residual weakness of his legs as a problem in that he was unable to keep up with his family when they went shopping together. Still another man with a similar degree of weakness was not as concerned about his ambulation but was particularly concerned that he no longer felt able to go fishing in a boat. Still another, with a similar level and degree of weakness, was far more concerned with the abnormal appearance of his gait; he was concerned about having to use a cane or otherwise appearing impaired, and his disability arose out of his sense of being different from his appearance prior to injury.

Although the neurological findings were similar in each case, the significance of those findings to each individual was unique. The degree to which each saw himself as impaired also, of course, differed in light of each person's own sense of self. The success of a restorative program would depend on the extent that it helped them to deal with their own, sometimes idiosyncratic, difficulties. By identifying the problem in terms that are meaningful to the individual, each person can participate in setting goals he is most likely committed to achieving.

A disability is thus defined to a much greater degree by the patient in the course of interviewing, and cannot be determined by the health professional on an a priori basis. One can determine the patient's impairments via the neurological examination even when the patient is comatose; one cannot make a determination of his disabilities without his active participation. The neurological examination seeks to determine objective data, but the search for definition of the disabilities must lead to the production of subjective data.

Along with the goal of minimizing a disability arising out of sensory or motor impairment, such as that of mobility, the restorative process must also prepare the person to enter into the third and most lasting stage: continuing care. A disabled person is not ordinarily an "ill" person merely by nature of continued disability. Yet there is a far higher likelihood of illness if the person with SCI does not carry out good health practices. The maintenance of his health requires a high degree of independent action, with ideally rare and short-lived interaction with health professionals.

This self-management includes the ability to identify the criteria to be used for the presence or absence of "health," generally in collaboration with the health professional. For example, since there is an increased likelihood of difficulties with the urinary tract, each person needs to develop some way to identify changes in his urine. Options include the color, odor, amount of sediment, or pH analogous to the methods used to measure glucosuria, or changes in body temperature or in urinary frequency.

The characteristics of "spinal man" frequently bring about not only an increase in the severity and incidence of specific illnesses but some modification in the effects of any disease process. It is important to develop those criteria that are specific to the individual. For example, the "normal" body temperature of a person with SCI may vary with the level of his neurological lesion and thus the significance of temperature as an indicator of infection will vary as well.

Another example arises out of the increased incidence in those with paraplegia of recurrent fractures in bones that have become osteoporotic due to lack of weight-bearing. The mode of presentation of fractures will also vary from the usual in persons with SCI. The signals of fracture

TABLE 1-1. *Information Gathering Process in SCI to Define the Problem*

Stage	Physician	Patient	Goals
Acute care	Asks the question via the neurological examination; focuses on the signs	Relatively passive	To determine the impairments
Rehabilitation	Asks the question via an interview; focuses on the symptoms	Collaborative	To determine the disabilities
Continuing care	—	Independent; asks the question of oneself using criteria previously established	To determine state of health; to decide when to seek professional care

are often idiosyncratic to the individual. An increase in one person's usual level of "spasticity" may be the signal or, in another, the evidence of illness will be swelling in a joint. Health professionals must greatly rely on the patient to provide such information about his or her own bodily reactions. Their goal is to enable the person to become better able to fulfill that role by helping him to define such criteria.

Although one may collaboratively establish the criteria as to when to seek medical help, evaluation must go on independently on a day-to-day basis. Lesser degrees of disturbance of function must also provide signals that the person with SCI should act to alleviate a problem. For example, many persons with SCI increase their fluid intake, and thus their urinary output, on the basis of those signals of urinary tract infection that they have come to use. One such person would act to increase his urinary output whenever he noted sweating and headache just prior to micturition. The aim of the health professional is to maintain and increase this ability to self-monitor on an ongoing basis and to act as an independent problem solver as well as to seek advice when appropriate.

Table 1-1 summarizes the patient–physician interaction at the three stages of care and the goals of the information collection procedures.

REFERENCES

1. Young JS, Burns PE, Bowen AM, McCutchen R (1982): *Spinal Cord Injury Statistics: Experience of the Regional Spinal Cord Injury Systems.* Phoenix: Good Samaritan Medical Center.

2. Guttmann L (1973): *Spinal Cord Injuries: Comprehensive Management and Research.* London: Blackwell Scientific Publishers.
3. Bedbrook G (1979): Spinal injuries with tetraplegia and paraplegia. *J Bone Joint Surg [Br]* 61:267.
4. Braakman R, Penning L (1971): *Injuries of the Cervical Spine.* Princeton, NJ: Excerpta Medica.
5. Bohlman H (1974): Traumatic fractures of the upper thoracic spine with paralysis: a study of 180 cases. *J Bone Joint Surg [Am]* 56:1299.
6. Haymaker W (1956): *Bing's Local Diagnosis in Neurological Diseases.* St. Louis: C.V. Mosby.
7. Heppenstall RB (1980): *Fracture Treatment and Healing.* Philadelphia: W. B. Saunders.
8. Stover SL, Fine PR, Go BK, et al. (1966): *Spinal Cord Injury: The Facts and Figures.* Birmingham, AL: University of Alabama at Birmingham.
9. Hussey R (1977): Problem-oriented medical record: a predetermined problem list for spinal cord injury. *Arch Phys Med Rehab* 58:314.
10. Wood PH, Bailey EM (1980): *People with Disabilities.* New York: World Rehabilitation Fund.
11. Fordyce W (1964): Personality characteristics in men with spinal cord injury as related to the manner of onset of injury. *Arch Phys Med Rehab* 45: 321–325.
12. Finkelstein V (1980): *Attitudes and Disabled People: Issues for Discussion.* New York: World Rehabilitation Fund, Monograph 5.
13. Fine P, DeVivo M, Go B, Lazarus P, Kartus P, Rutt B, Stover S (1985): The state of the national SCI database. *Paraplegia* 12:51–52.
14. Borges P, Hackler R (1982): The urologic status of the Vietnam War paraplegic: a 15 year follow-up. *J Urol* 127:710–711.

CHAPTER 2
Acute Care

The goals of the acute care phase are, in order of priority, to stabilize vital signs, to minimize further injury to the spinal cord, and to initiate the restorative process. This chapter will focus on medical and surgical interventions specific to the character of the injury to the spinal cord and its ligamentous and osseous supports, with the understanding that maintenance of adequate ventilation and circulatory status is primary. Stabilizing the support system to protect the spinal cord from further neurological impairment or to enhance possible return of function is the major objective. In this context, there remains the goal of early mobilization of the patient to speed rehabilitation and prevent the medical complications leading to morbidity and even mortality. Figure 2-1 describes an order of planning for the total management of the newly injured person (1).

THE NATURE OF THE INJURY

Neurological aspects

Data concerning the site and extent of damage to the nervous system provide the primary basis for clinical decision-making during this stage. Examination of motor, sensory, reflex, and autonomic functions is ongoing, and judgment must be made as to the level of injury to the spinal cord (longitudinal) and its degree of completeness (transverse). The determination of the level of injury is crucial so that proper radiological or other imaging examination can be made. Ongoing monitoring provides data as to need for surgical intervention and a basis for planning rehabilitation. A more global measure of neurological impairment may also be used to statistically evaluate the effectiveness of specific management programs.

The degree of longitudinal involvement is determined by the lowest level at which there is both normal motor and sensory function. The

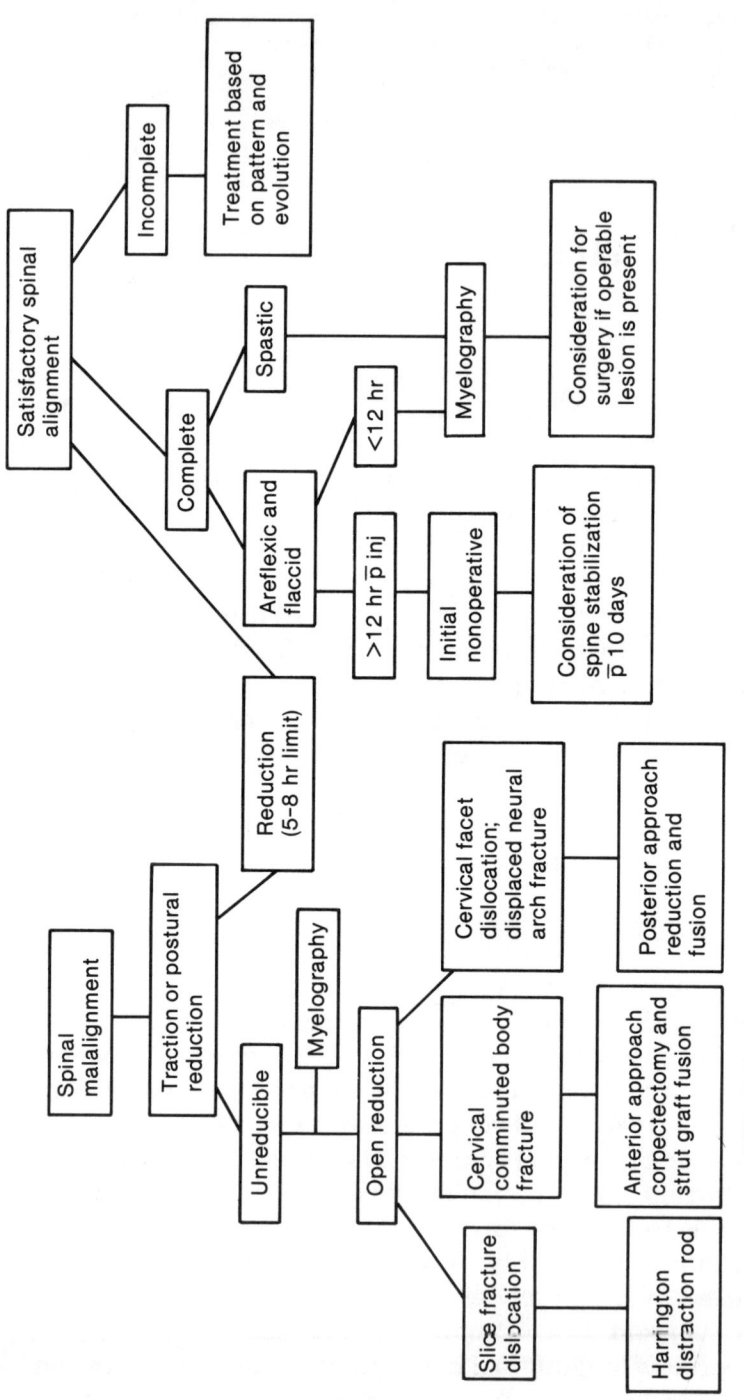

FIG. 2-1. Management in the early post-injury phase. (Reproduced by permission from ref. 1.)

TABLE 2-1. *Key Muscles for Motor Level Classification*

C4:	Diaphragm
C5:	Deltoid and/or biceps
C6:	Wrist extensors
C7:	Triceps
C8:	Flexor profundus
T1:	Hand instrinsics
T2-L1:	Use sensory level, abdominal reflexes, and Beevor's sign to help localize lowest normal neurological segment
L2:	Iliopsoas
L3:	Quadriceps
L4:	Tibialis anterior
L5:	Extensor hallucis longus
S1:	Gastrocnemius
S2-S5:	Use sensory level

normal motor neurological level is considered the lowest intact segment in which the muscle grade is at least "fair" (3/5), with active movement through the range of motion against gravity (2). Key muscles for motor level determination are listed in Table 2-1. A motor score index useful for ongoing evaluation is derived by examining the 10 bilateral muscles, excluding the diaphragm. There is a total potential score of 100 using the scoring system for each muscle, in which 0 = total paralysis; 1 = palpable or visible contraction; 2 = active movement through full range of motion (ROM) with gravity eliminated; 3 = active movement through ROM against gravity; 4 = active movement through ROM against resistance; and 5 = normal. The key indicators using the sensory dermatomes are listed in Table 2-2.

During the early post-injury phase, the deep and superficial reflexes are generally abolished below the level of the lesion. This "spinal shock" may last from several days to up to 6 weeks (4). The lowest reflexes reappear first: the anal wink and bulbocavernosus reflexes. The return or continued presence of these reflexes in the post-injury phase indicates integrity of the sacral cord segments (S2-S4). The bulbocavernosus reflex is elicited by compression of the glans penis (or clitoris) or other stimulus in the same afferent segment (tugs on an indwelling catheter), with consequent contraction of the external sphincter of the anus felt by the inserted index finger (5). The anal wink is a contraction of the anal sphincter following local stimulation in the anus or the perianal region.

Vasomotor disturbances of spinal origin do not have as clear-cut a segmental distribution as the motor and sensory functions, although there is some localizing value within the thoracolumbar sympathetic outflow. For example, the spinal vasomotor (and sudomotor) center for

TABLE 2-2. *Sensory Dermatomes for Classification of Level**

Cervical segments
    C5:   Anterolateral shoulder
    C6:   Thumb
    C7:   Middle finger
    C8:   Little finger
Thoracic segments
    T1:   Medial arm
    T3:   3rd, 4th interspace
    T4:   Nipple line, 4th-5th interspace
    T6:   Xiphoid
    T10: Navel
    T12: Pubis
Lumbar segments
    L2:   Medial thigh
    L3:   Medial knee
    L4:   Medial ankle, great toe
    L5:   Dorsum of foot
Sacral segments
    S1:   Lateral foot
    S2:   Posterolateral thigh
    S3-S5: Perianal area

*Adapted from ref. 3.

the head and neck and heart is in segment T1-T4; for the upper limb in T2-T7; and for the lower limb in T10-L1. An injury to the midthoracic cord may therefore give rise to cyanosis and anhidrosis of the upper limb without altering motor or sensory function in that same limb (6). Clinically significant sympathetic dysfunction manifests itself as an inability to increase cardiac output via an increase in pulse rate. Ongoing vagal tone arising from the intact parasympathetic system produces a relative bradycardia in those with a lesion above T1.

The extent of involvement of the sympathetic outflow along the course of the thoracic cord determines the degree to which the person has become poikilothermic. Paralysis of sweating and vasomotor control of the skin increases the likelihood of hyperthermia as the lesion increasingly involves segments of the cord from T8 upward. Lower thoracic segments are the source of fibers carried by the splanchnic nerve involved in the maintenance of blood pressure and responsiveness to change in position. T5 is the most cranial segment participating in the maintenance of vasomotor control within the abdominal vessels. Lesions above that level can lead not only to orthostatic hypotension but also to the later development of autonomic hyper-reflexia (7) (to be discussed more fully later in this volume).

Bilateral damage to the spinal cord at or above the level of the sacral outflow (S2-S5) manifests itself in parasympathetic dysfunction. Urinary and fecal retention is due to loss, at least initially, of the contraction of the walls of the bladder (and rectum) and the coordinated relaxation of the equivalent sphincters. Cholinergic innervation of the bladder smooth muscle is via the pelvic nerves that originate in the grey matter of the sacral cord segments S2-S4 (detrusor nucleus). Adrenergic innervation is via the hypogastric nerve from spinal cord segment T11-T12. The pudendal nerves innervate the external urethral sphincter and arise from ventral sacral roots S2-S4.

The most obvious effects on sexual function are on erection in the male. In the early stages, there is loss of both "reflexogenic" erections secondary to penile stimulation due to disruption of the sacral parasympathetic outflow and loss of "psychogenic" erections due to disconnection from the high lumbar sympathetic outflow. In complete lesions, the penis may become enlarged due to passive engorgement of the corpora cavernosa secondary to paralytic dilatation of the vasoconstrictor fibers in the sympathetic system (7). True priapism in the early phase requires persistence of partial conduction or an "incomplete" injury.

Traumatic injury to the sacral cord is usually associated with concomitant injury to the lumbar roots. The conus medullaris syndrome is defined by an areflexic bladder, bowel, and lower extremities, with absence of the bulbocavernosus reflex. In those rare instances when the conus alone is injured, the lower extremities are free of motor disturbance, since they derive almost their entire innervation from segments above the conus. Cauda equina syndrome due to injury to the lumbar roots existing from the spinal cord below the level of the conus may manifest findings similar to those of the conus itself. Differential diagnosis is aided by asymmetrical findings in root involvement (6). There are also implications for return of function for those impairments resulting from root involvement per se (8).

Knowledge of the longitudinal level of injury is useful for planning in terms of expected disability. The major categories that define functional consequences are quadriparesis or quadriplegia versus paraparesis or paraplegia. More specific relationships between the level of injury and the functional consequences are described in later chapters. In addition, determination of the degree of completeness of the transverse extent of the injury is particularly helpful in predicting improvement in the degree of expected impairment. A prime goal of this early phase is to protect the spinal cord to enhance such improvement, with surgical intervention as needed.

The "zone of injury" (2) consists of up to three neurological segments

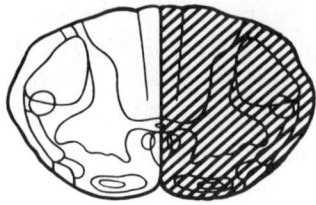

FIG. 2-2. Brown-Sequard syndrome. Modified hemisection of cord. Homolateral paralysis and contralateral sensory loss. (Reproduced by permission from ref. 28.)

at the point of damage to the spinal cord. There may be some preservation of motor and/or sensory function within this area, although activity may reflect involvement of the roots rather than the spinal cord itself. A "complete" injury is reflected by the absence of any motor and/or sensory function below the level of the zone of injury, while an "incomplete" one, with less than complete physiological transection of the cord, is characterized by preservation of function below the level of the zone of injury, including sacral sparing. Any continued conduction within the spinal cord has major significance for later improvement (9).

Any return of reflex activity (signifying abatement of spinal shock) below the level of the lesion, but without return of motor or sensory function, has a poor prognosis for future recovery, indicating that the cord segment and the nerve roots controlling that reflex are intact and that the distal segments have been isolated from the brain (8).

Anatomical classification of incomplete injuries, in order of decreasing prognosis for significant neurological recovery, consist of 1) Brown-Sequard syndrome (Fig. 2-2), 2) central cervical cord syndrome (Fig. 2-3), 3) anterior cord syndrome (Fig. 2-4), and 4) posterior cord syndrome (Fig. 2-5).

Mixed syndromes are not uncommon. A more functional classification of impairment is that of Frankel et al. (10), which has been used for the statistical evaluation of patient care programs. Complete injuries are graded as "A." Incomplete injuries are graded "B" if there is preservation of sensation only, "C" if there is any preservation of nonfunctional motor function, and "D" if there is any preservation of functional motor action. The "E" category signifies complete return of motor and sensory function even if abnormal reflexes remain.

FIG. 2-3. Central cord syndrome. Dissociation in degree of motor weakness with lower limbs stronger than upper limbs and sacral sensory sparing. (Reproduced by permission from ref. 28.)

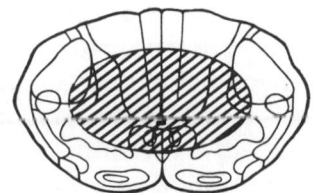

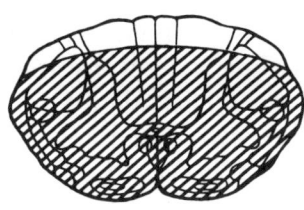

FIG. 2-4. Anterior cord syndrome. Motor paralysis with hypesthesia, hypalgesia, and preservation of posterior column sensory function. (Reproduced by permission from ref. 28.)

Orthopedic aspects

The extent of injury to the osseus-ligamentous support of the spinal cord has major implications for management in the acute phase, given the goal of minimizing impairment and enabling early mobilization. The presence of fracture(s) and the degree of malalignment of the vertebrae are generally determined by plain radiography or computed tomography (CT), measuring the degree of separation of the spinous processes, and the anteroposterior displacement of the vertebrae and the degree of angulation. Malalignment of the spinal elements reduces the capacity of the spinal canal and should be alleviated as promptly as possible to prevent further impairment. Skeletal traction with tongs or via halo to the skull can begin immediately for those with cervical spine injuries. If external traction is ineffective, open reduction and stabilization of the spine via fusion is carried out. See Hussey et al. (1) for a description of a general plan of action.

Once alignment has been achieved, the issue of decompression must be addressed. The finding of an incomplete injury increases the possible value of decompression in maximizing opportunity for improvement. The indications for decompression are quite limited. If improvement is steady and rapid, as determined by serial neurological examinations, intervention need not be contemplated as in the Brown-Sequard and central cord syndromes. CT with or without myelography is done if an early plateau is not followed by further improvement on neurological examination, in order to demonstrate bone or disc fragments suitable for surgical removal. The surgical approach is determined by the site of the impingement. An anterior surgical approach (with fusion) is used when there are findings of anterior impingement on the cord. Evi-

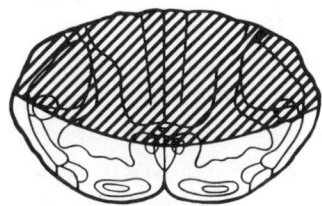

FIG. 2-5. Posterior cord syndrome. Motor paralysis with loss of posterior column sensory function (very rare). (Reproduced by permission from ref. 28.)

dence of neurological deterioration plus the finding of an epidural hematoma on myelography constitutes the rare occasion when laminectomy is called for. This same posterior surgical approach would also be used for findings of posterior impingement by bone fragments on the spinal cord.

Once alignment has been achieved and the need for decompression (with fusion) excluded, the likelihood of stable healing must be determined. Unstable injuries may not only jeopardize the spinal cord and roots in the acute phase but also lead to later instability with pain and/or neurological deterioration. The alternatives are either surgical stabilization, generally posterior fusion, as soon as medical stabilization has occurred, orthotic stabilization such as the halo-brace, or bedrest with or without skeletal traction. Early surgical stabilization has been a controversial area [see Bedbrook (11)]. The standard method of treatment for cervical spine injuries in most parts of the world is nonsurgical stabilization with tongs in place and traction maintained on a bed that permits frequent turning. The increasing use in the United States of a halo with vest, particularly for injuries in the area of C6 or above, permits earlier mobilization than the several months required with nonsurgical stabilization.

It is important to recognize that there is a spectrum of "instability." The determination of the degree of instability depends on the radiographic findings as well as the likely mechanism of injury, the pattern of fracture, and history (12). For example, a history of a progressive neurological deficit or spine deformity is indicative of instability until proved otherwise. Radiographic findings indicating instability of the cervical spine show angulation of greater than 11° and/or greater than 3.5 mm displacement of the vertebral body (13). A more complete method for the determination of clinical instability in the lower cervical spine is that of White et al. (14).

Disruption to the posterior ligamentous complex with involvement of the disc is considered to be the major basis of instability. Particular mechanisms of injury lead to such a pattern, and the likely mechanism of injury can often be deduced from the history and the location of associated injuries. Instability in the cervical area occurs when flexion or extension is combined with axial loading, as in diving mishaps and in automobile accidents that involve the head hitting the windshield. The addition of a rotational component with flexion is particularly likely to lead to instability (13). At least one generally accepted protocol recommends posterior fusion as an elective procedure even when, in the instance of bilateral facet dislocation, closed reduction had been successful and the option was available for the use of a halo-jacket for immobilization of the spine (15).

If, in evaluating instability, evidence of bony involvement or displacement on the static X-ray films could not account for the neurological findings, a stretch test with traction on a cervical halter may identify underlying ligamentous damage, which may limit stable healing. Any change in neurological status, an interspace separation of greater than 1.7 mm, or any angulation greater than 7.5°, is considered positive evidence. If these studies still have not identified the cause of the neurological involvement, consideration may be given to the use of flexion–extension views (15).

The management of injuries to the upper thoracic spine (T1-T10) to achieve stable healing differs from that of the cervical spine. Fractures to the thoracic spine are reasonably stable because the surrounding rib cage acts like a splint. However, serious ligamentous injuries occur and lead to instability with late deformity. Severe kyphosis can result, particularly secondary to the use of laminectomy. Postural traction with hyperextension in a turning bed is generally used for up to 6–8 weeks with subsequent chest orthosis. Surgical stabilization is not generally required unless a total dislocation exists (16).

The analysis of the degree of mechanical instability in the thoracic and thoracolumbar spine is based on a modification of the Holdsworth classification (15). In this "three-column" theory, instability requires the rupture of at least both the posterior column (pedicles, facet joints, spinous processes, and interspinous and supraspinous ligaments) and the middle column (posterior longitudinal ligament, posterior annulus fibrosis, and posterior half of vertebral body). The anterior column consists of the anterior longitudinal ligament, anterior portion of the annulus, and the anterior half of the vertebral body (15).

Injuries to the thoracolumbar junction (T10-L1) are much more likely to be unstable than those of the upper thoracic spine, and all such injuries should be considered as unstable initially (16). The use of open reduction and internal fixation by Harrington rods with bony fusion (17) is increasingly accepted. This is done as soon as possible to permit early mobilization in a body jacket, thus shortening the total rehabilitation time.

The management of the osseus-ligamentous aspects of SCI varies widely with the level, type, and severity of injury. The spine repairs itself by healing the disrupted ligaments, by repairing the fracture site itself, or by spontaneous fusion between injured vertebrae (18). The healing of torn ligaments leads to replacement by fibrous tissue, which is often not as strong as the original ligaments and is not sufficient to produce stability. Spontaneous fusion and normal fracture healing produces a more stable union. Thus, determining the degree of stability that may be expected and the necessity for surgical intervention is complex and depends on a variety of factors including the degree of bony versus ligamentous injury and the segment of the spine involved. The foregoing provides the reader with some of the general principles that underlie decisions in individual cases.

TREATMENT APPROACHES

The goals of treatment in the acute phase are to stabilize the person with SCI while minimizing neurological impairment, and to enable early mobilization while protecting the spine so that healing can occur without deformity. Once the character and degree of the neurological and osseus/ligamentous injury have been determined, a treatment program specific to the level and extent of the injury is instituted. The criteria for surgical intervention have already been described as well as some of the bases for the selection of any particular intervention. This section focuses on medical management, with particular emphasis on those aspects that are relatively unique to the character of the injury to the spinal cord and its supports.

Medical treatment to reduce the likelihood of damage to the spinal cord following trauma has been an area of increasing interest. The value of steroids has not been confirmed. Recent animal studies suggest that opiate antagonists and/or TRH may prove clinically useful (19).

Although not specific to SCI, one of the major causes of morbidity and mortality in the acute phase is deep vein thrombosis with subsequent pulmonary embolus and infarction (20). Recent studies have shown the value of low dose heparin with ergotamine in reducing the frequency of this complication in postoperative patients, with possible extrapolation to persons with SCI (22).

Heterotopic ossification (HO) rather than deep vein thrombosis may be the source of the swelling and erythema in the extremities below the level of the lesion (21). Positive findings in the early phase of the three-phase bone scan may identify the existence of HO prior to visualization on radiography. Etidronate suppresses bone turnover and may retard mineralization of the osteoid formed outside the articular surface. It may thus reduce the inflammatory response to calcification and reduce the likelihood of later problems with range of motion of the affected limbs.

Treatment procedures during the acute phase provide a transition to the restorative phase. They deal with the continued stabilization during the weeks-long healing process; the prevention of contractures and other deformities that may interfere with mobility; and the prevention of further impairment of the function of the skin and the urinary and gastrointestinal systems. The treatment program lays the groundwork for both later rehabilitation and the even later continuing care phase for health maintenance.

The stabilization of those patients who have undergone surgery as well as those for whom surgery had not been indicated generally requires the use of orthotic devices, which immobilize the spinal column and aid in healing, to permit relative mobility and participation in active rehabilitation. The terminology that describes these devices uses the initial English term for the joints to be encompassed. For example, in some settings, following surgical fusion in the cervical area, a head cervical orthosis such as the Philadelphia collar may be used. For others, a head cervical thoracic orthosis encompassing these several joints may be indicated. Still others may have a halo-vest skeletal traction used to immobilize the cervical spine, even after surgery for fusion. For those thoracolumbar injuries with internal fixation, a molded body jacket might be used. See Redford (23) for a full discussion of the available alternatives.

The selection of an orthosis and the time during which it is applied is affected by the degree of osseous versus ligamentous injury and other factors as described above. The removal of the external support, after some weeks or months, depends on evidence of stability as indicated on flexion–extension films of the areas of the spine involved.

During the early period post-injury, deep tendon reflexes are absent or depressed during the period of "spinal shock." Its physiological basis has been attributed to the sudden loss of the predominantly facilitatory influence of the descending supraspinal tracts, with a specific effect on the gamma motor neurons in the anterior horns (4). The relaxation of the intrafusal fibers leads to reduction in the stimuli entering the spindles, with a subsequent effect on reflex stimulation. Although the more caudal reflexes may begin to return within as short a time as 24 hours, the extent of the spinal shock and its duration varies considerably, ranging for up to 6 weeks. In general, reflexes that remain absent to the greatest degree are those closest to the level of the lesion. The duration is shortened by freedom from sepsis, due most frequently to urinary tract infection, pressure sores, and respiratory infections.

Although the neurological impairment may remain fixed during this acute phase, proper management can help to minimize the eventual effects on function of those impairments. The goals are to establish the optimal conditions for the return of activity in the bowels, bladder, and the respiratory and other skeletal muscles.

Ventilatory impairment is one of the most serious complications leading to morbidity and mortality during this early phase (24). Impaired inspiration with a lesion at C4 affecting the diaphragm requires ventilator support. In general, ventilator support is necessary if the pCO_2 is over 40 or the pO_2 is below 60. Those with lower cervical or high thoracic lesions have impaired action of the intercostal and abdominal muscles, with effects, respectively, on both inspiration and expiration. Expiratory reserve is particularly affected, with a loss of the ability to cough and thus to clear secretions. In those with sympathetic denervation of the heart, reflex bradycardia with or without cardiac arrest is particularly likely following tracheal stimulation when hypoxia is present. The unopposed vagal action may require the use of atropine as well as adequate oxygenation before tracheal suctioning.

Active pulmonary toilet, including postural drainage, is necessary for the prevention of atelectasis and infection. Incentive spirometry can provide an ongoing training tool to encourage deep breathing by providing immediate visual feedback. Assisted cough by applying extrinsic pressure to abdominal contents ("quad cough") is a useful skill. An abdominal binder helps those with weakened diaphragmatic excursion to support their abdominal contents while sitting. The binder prevents the weakened abdominal muscles from causing a decrease in abdominal visceral hydrostatic pressure by increasing the recoil and inspiratory excursion of the diaphragm and thus vital capacity (25).

Although the level of impairment may remain, vital capacity increases after the spinal shock phase. An increase in the activity of newly recruited accessory muscles such as the sternocleidomastoid and trapezius may occur above the level of the lesion. However, with the return of "tone," the act of breathing itself apparently serves as an appropriate stimulus, evoking a stretch reflex with subsequent increased activity in the intercostal muscles even below the level of the lesion (4).

The effects of "spinal shock" are not limited to the striated muscles. During the acute phase, the urinary bladder no longer responds to an appropriate degree of distension by efficient contraction of the detrusor muscles. There is a flaccid paralysis of the smooth muscles in the wall of the bladder and a paralysis of the bladder neck innervated by the sympathetic and parasympathetic systems and the striated urinary sphincter in the urethra. Retention of urine occurs, and voiding takes place through overflow when the intravesicular pressure is high enough to overcome the paralyzed sphincter. Long-standing atonicity of the bladder wall will result if overdistension is permitted (over 500 ml), and the bladder wall will not be as effective in emptying once the spinal shock has ended. An indwelling catheter is used in the emergency situation, after which intermittent catheterization is started on a regular schedule to prevent overdistension. Initially, intermittent catheterization should be done on a 4-hour basis, with appropriate restriction of fluid intake to prevent overdistension between catheterizations. The eventual character of the bladder management program depends on whether the level of lesion is at the sacral outflow or above and will be discussed more fully later in this volume.

Paralysis of peristalsis is accompanied by ileus and fecal retention, particularly in those with upper thoracic or cervical lesions. Bowel sounds are absent or markedly diminished. Such paralysis may also affect the stomach, producing gastric dilatation and subsequent interference with ventilatory capacity. Like those of micturition, the reflexes controlling defecation are also abolished during spinal shock. Protection against these effects requires decompression of the bowels and, following the return of peristalsis, the development of a reflex bowel evacuation program. Evacuation can occur using suppositories, which stimulate reflex activity, as well as bowel softeners and dietary bulk early on. Like bladder management, the character of the bowel program will vary depending on whether the lesion is at the level of the sacral cord or above (7).

Perhaps the most debilitating and frequently the most costly consequences of spinal shock that affect active participation in rehabilitation are pressure sores. During this early phase, "lying down" sores occur in the sacrum and heels, particularly in those with complete quadriplegia. Loss of vasomotor tone in the skin due to denervation of the sympathetic outflow increases the likelihood of pressure ischemia. Skin over bony parts close to the surface is more likely to be affected. Pressure is relieved by turning the patient frequently, generally at 2-hour intervals, and by paying particular attention to proper padding and positioning of bony prominences (7).

The prevention of muscle contracture at the joints also helps to minimize functional loss despite the continuation of the neurological impairment. Such contractures could cause pain later as well as interfere with motor actions. Particularly important is the prevention of unopposed flexion. In the past, prolonged fixation of the paralyzed lower limbs in adduction and semi-flexion by placement of pillows under the knees led to later paralysis-in-flexion, limiting the ability to sit as well as presenting general problems in nursing care. Treatment consists of maintaining, while supine, abduction and extension at the hips and knees, and keeping feet and toes dorsiflexed; positioning in the prone position to the extent possible; and early passive movements of the paralyzed limbs through their full range of motion (7). Some joints may require even greater range of motion than normal. For example, the long sitting position used during dressing by a person with paraplegia requires 110° of hip flexion.

In the upper extremities, it is particularly important to maintain a full range of shoulder motion for use later in propelling a wheelchair. In those with quadriplegia, positioning the arms in 90° of abduction for 1–2 hours several times each day is recommended to prevent painful shoulder contracture later. In those with involvement at the level of C5, prevention of flexion deformity due to the unopposed action of the elbow flexors will maintain the option for later surgery and the transfer of a portion of the deltoid to regain elbow extension (26). The action of the wrist and fingers must be maintained to permit their use later in gripping. Coordinated finger flexion and wrist extension—the tenodesis hand—is usually sought for those with lesions at the level of C6.

During this early phase of spinal shock, it is particularly important (Parks H., personal communication) to maintain the full range of motion at the joints despite the changes in vascular tone that may have occurred with swelling of the soft tissue. Pain that might limit passive movement through the full range of motion should be treated with anti-inflammatory agents or analgesics.

REFERENCES

1. Hussey R, Rossier A, Sarkarati M (1983): An algorithm or treatment plan for acute spinal cord injury. *Am Paraplegia Soc* 6:27.
2. American Spinal Injury Association (1984): *Standards for Neurological Classification of Spinal Injury Patients.* Chicago: American Spinal Injury Association.
3. Donovan WH, Bedbrook G (1982): *Comprehensive Management of Spinal Cord Injury.* Summit, NJ: Ciba-Geigy, Ciba Symposium 34:2.
4. Guttman L (1976): Spinal shock. In: *Handbook of Clinical Neurology: Injuries of the Spine and Spinal Cord, Part II,* vol 26, edited by Vinkar PJ, Bruyn GW. Amsterdam: North Holland Publishing, pp 243–262.
5. Bors E, French J (1952): Management of paroxysmal hypertension following injuries to the cervical and upper thoracic segments of spinal cord. 64:803.

6. Haymaker W (1956): *Bing's Local Diagnosis in Neurological Diseases.* St Louis: C.V. Mosby.
7. Guttmann L (1973): *Spinal Cord Injuries: Comprehensive Management and Research.* London: Blackwell Scientific Publishers.
8. Holdworth FW (1970): Fractures, dislocations, and fracture-dislocations of the spine. *J Bone Joint Surg [Br]* 52:1534.
9. Klose K, Goldberg M, Smith R, Green B (1980): Neurological change following spinal cord injury: an assessment technique and preliminary results. *Sci Digest* 2:35–42.
10. Frankel H, Hancock D, Hyslop G, Melzak J, Michaels L, Ungar G, Vernon J, Walsh J (1969): The value of postural reduction in the initial management of closed injuries to the spine with paraplegia and tetraplegia. *Paraplegia* 7:179–192.
11. Bedbrook G (1979): Spinal injuries with tetraplegia and paraplegia. *J Bone Joint Surg* 61B:267.
12. Gertzbein S (1982): Assessment of cervical spine instability. In: *Early Management of Acute Spinal Cord Injury,* edited by Tator CH. New York: Raven Press, pp 41–52.
13. Heppenstall RB (1980): *Fracture Treatment and Healing.* Philadelphia: W.B. Saunders.
14. White A, Southwick W, Panjabi M (1976): Clinical instability in lower cervical spine: a review of past and current concepts. *Spine* 1:15.
15. American Academy of Orthopedic Surgeons (1984): *Orthopedic Update.* Chicago: American Academy of Orthopedic Surgeons.
16. Bohlman H (1974): Traumatic fractures of the upper thoracic spine with paralysis: a study of 180 cases. *J Bone Joint Surg [Am]* 56:1299.
17. Ahn J, Ragnarrson K, Gordon W, Goldfinger G, Lewin A (1984): Current trends in stabilizing high thoracic and thoracolumbar spine fractures. *Arch Phys Med Rehab* 65:366.
18. Hussey RW (1982): Spinal cord injury. In: *Orthopedic Rehabilitation,* edited by Nickel VL. New York: Churchill Livingstone.
19. Fader A, Jacobs T, Smith M, Holaday J (1983): Comparison of thyrotropin-releasing hormone (TRH), naloxone and decamethasone treatment in experimental spinal cord injury. *Neurology* 33:673.
20. Young JS, Burns PE, Bowen AM, McCutchen R (1982): *Spinal Cord Injury Statistics: Experience of the Regional Spinal Cord Injury Systems.* Phoenix: Good Samaritan Medical Center.
21. Stover SL, Hataway CJ, Zeiger HE (1975): Heterotopic ossification in spinal cord-injured patients. *Arch Phys Med Rehab* 56:199–204.
22. Sasahara A, DiSerio F, Singer J (1984): Dihydroergotamine-heparin prophylaxis of postoperative deep vein thrombosis. *AMA* 251:2690.
23. Redford JB (1987): Orthotics. In: *Physical Medicine and Rehabilitation State of the Art Reviews,* vol 1, no 1. Philadelphia: Hanley and Belfus.
24. Fiegl-Meyer A (1976): The respiratory system. In: *Handbook of Clinical*

Neurology: Injuries of the Spine and Spinal Cord, Part II, vol 26, edited by Vinkar PJ, Bruyn GW. Amsterdam: North Holland Publishing, pp 335–349.
25. Saltzstein R, Melvin J (1986): Ventilatory compromise in SCI: a review. *J Am Paraplegia Soc* 9:6–9.
26. Moberg E (1975): Surgical treatment for absent single-hand grip and elbow extension in quadriplegia. *J Bone Joint Surg [Am]* 57:196–206.
27. Pavlakis A, Siroky M, Goldstein I, Krane R (1983): Neurological findings in conus medullaris and cauda equina injury. *Arch Neurol* 40:570–573.
28. American Spinal Injury Association (1984): *Standards for Neurological Classification of Spinal Injury Patients.* Chicago: ASIA, p. 5.

CHAPTER 3

Rehabilitation

In contrast to the acute care phase, during which every attempt is made to minimize further injury to the spinal cord, the overall goal of the rehabilitation phase is to minimize the disabilities created by the neurological impairments, although the latter may continue to exist. These disabilities include effects on life activities brought about by the loss of nervous system functions heretofore available. Their minimization requires enhancing those abilities that remain unimpaired and developing additional or alternative methods of accomplishing life activities.

Adjustments are usually required in the ways one accomplishes tasks. It is frequently necessary to help the person with SCI to reorganize ways of thinking so that he or she can become clearer about the goals or outcomes being sought and differentiate between these outcomes and the methods or actions by which they can be achieved. The outcomes one seeks may or may not remain the same as before the injury. The ability to maintain mobility remains a goal, but the methods for reaching this outcome must usually change. Ambulation, for example, may no longer be available as a means of achieving mobility.

The person with SCI must also recognize that alternative methods for the accomplishment of goals do exist, and that they are not necessarily *worse* by virtue of being *different*. The "normal" method—that which is perhaps used by most or that which had been the usual method for that person before injury—is not the *only* method. For example, it may be helpful to recognize that even before injury, ambulation was never the sole means of achieving mobility, or perhaps even the most commonly used one given the availability of wheeled conveyances.

The person with SCI must not only reorganize his thinking but, in many instances, must become far better organized in it than in the past. Alternative methods of accomplishing tasks generally require far more conscious planning and monitoring. What was lost are those inputs to which the person had responded unconsciously as well as ingrained ways of responding. The brain—that portion of the nervous system that remains unimpaired—must be used to develop the necessary alternative methods.

One aim of rehabilitation is therefore education—to learn new ways to carry out crucial life tasks. Learning new methods frequently requires the use of cognition and planning, skills that may not be fully developed in the person who most often incurs a spinal cord injury, given his average level of education and relative youth. It is thus frequently necessary not only to learn new ways of doing things but also to make a commitment to a process of injury by which one may continue to discover new ways of achieving one's goals after injury.

Rehabilitation is thus based on a planning process detailed in Chapter 5. One aim of an effective planning process is the setting of clear goals and their eventual accomplishment using means that may differ from those used prior to injury. Still another aim is to learn how to plan for oneself. This experience during the rehabilitation phase provides the basis for active participation in the management of one's continuing care in changing circumstances.

IMPAIRMENTS AND DISABILITIES

The determination of impairments for the purpose of establishing a rehabilitation plan differs from the neurological examination, used primarily to localize neurological disease. For example, although impaired motor actions are most obvious on examination and are frequently most helpful for localizing the level of injury, they are not necessarily most serious in terms of functional effects. Moberg (1) has properly emphasized that "useful" motor actions are secondary in that they are responses to afferent inputs, which he considers primary. The example is given of the driver who carries out the appropriate motor action only after seeing an approaching car to which he must yield. Even more serious are the functional effects of the isolation of the thoracolumbar and sacral autonomic outflow of the spinal cord from its supraspinal connections. The neurological examination as related to rehabilitation issues must reflect these factors.

Goal setting is an important part of the rehabilitation process. Disabilities—the person's real-life problems—must be determined in order to set appropriate goals. The character of the disability—the functional consequences in life terms—is determined to a major degree but not entirely by the kind and degree of neurological impairment. The major disabilities are those that relate to "self-care" in those with impairments in the upper extremities, mobility in those with impairments in the lower extremities, and the control of perineal functions—defecation, urination, and sex—for all those with spinal cord injuries.

The significance of any particular loss of function will vary with individual priorities. For one person, the loss of mobility may be particularly significant, while for another the major problem will be the loss of previous methods of achieving sexual intimacy. Such priorities can obviously affect the design of the rehabilitation program.

The third component contributing to the nature of the disability is the environment in which the person with impairment lives: job requirements, the availability of caretakers, and the physical characteristics of the life space.

This section delineates the various impairments and the resulting disabilities associated with SCI and later describes the approaches to lessen the impact of those disabilities on the person's life.

Sensation

The receipt of adequate information is a crucial need that is disrupted by the neural disconnection in SCI. The loss of awareness of that portion of the body below the level of the lesion deprives the person of the input, ordinarily unconscious, that permits the constant monitoring and subsequent fine-tuning of motor actions. For example, a sense of discomfort can no longer be counted on to signal ischemia of the skin and muscles when sitting for long periods in one position, and it becomes necessary to develop a program for the relief of pressure. Instead of relying on the signals of ischemia, one may use a clock, which, at least initially, must actually be visualized. What has previously been a "closed loop" in which input to the central nervous system had brought about an adaptation without conscious awareness must now become an "open loop" in which, at least initially, a deliberate decision to act on conscious input must occur.

The determination of the type of sensory loss particularly significant to the disruption of function differs from the tests used in the neurological examination. The differential finding of impairments in terms of pinprick and temperature, touch with cotton wool, and viabratory sense with a tuning fork is useful in localizing lesions in the nervous system. Quite different, however, is the significant sensory finding in relation to function of the hand. In order to plan appropriately to reduce disability, Moberg (2) found the relevant afferent input to be that of "tactile gnosis"—the ability of the fingers and hand to "see" what they are doing. Being able to differentiate the two blunt ends of a paper clip less than 10 mm apart establishes the availability of cutaneous sensibility for learning and control. In its absence, visual input is the only alternative. A person dependent on vision can use only one hand at a time, which has significant implications for the choice of treatment to reduce the degree of disability in grasp and other hand actions.

Even when the modality tested is relevant to function—such as sharp pain when examined by pinprick—the neurological examination may fail to reflect the true situation. The absence of sensation to pinprick below the level of the lesion on standard testing during the neurological examination may not also be indicative of the absence of pain. The patient may feel pain when repeated stimuli are applied to several areas, inducing temporal or spatial summation. Sensations requiring more intense and prolonged stimulation reflect conduction within the slower unmyelinated fibers rather than the faster fibers that conduct pinprick. The awareness of pain may persist for several seconds, simulating the burning, relatively long-lasting, poorly localized chronic pain without any apparent source that is frequently disabling to persons with SCI (3).

A crucial aspect of the reorganization of the nervous system that goes on during rehabilitation relates to increased sensitivity to those inputs that can now serve as relatively consistent signals of danger or injury. For example, the diffuse burning sensation described above may serve to signal ischemia of the skin or muscle due to excessive unrelieved pressure. In the absence of the sensation of fullness of the bladder and/or rectum, some persons with lesions above T5 use the sympathetic discharge of sweating or a transient increase in cardiac output as a signal of distension and the need for evacuation.

Motor function

The determination of the motor impairments used for localization provides a useful, albeit sometimes gross, estimate of the subsequent functional disability (see Table 3-1). For example, the critical neurological level for functional independence in those with quadriplegia is C6 and C7. Those whose injury is at C4 or C5 will clearly require assistance in achieving life tasks with the upper limbs, those whose injury is at C8 should be capable of achieving independence in all self-care activities despite some impairment of the upper limbs, and those at the critical level of C6 and C7 are on the borderline of achieving total independence in self-care.

In a study of persons with injury at those levels living in the community, Welch et al. (4) sampled a wide range of activities including

REHABILITATION

TABLE 3-1. *Functional Goals by Level of Impairment**

Level	Mobility	Transfer†	ADL†	Dress†	Bowel care†	Bladder care†	Attendant care	Special equipment‡
C1-C2	Elec W/C	D	D	D	D	D	Full-time	Environmental control respirator
C3	Elec W/C	D	D	D	D	D	Full-time	Environmental control
C4	Elec W/C	D	D	D	D	D	Full-time	Environmental control
C5	Elec W/C	D	D	D	D	D	Full-time	Low eff steer
C6	Man W/C car	?IN	MA	?IN	D	D	Part-time	Adapted utensil and tenodesis splint
C7	Man W/C car	IN	IN	IN	D	A	Part-time	
C8	Man W/C car	IN	IN	IN	A	MA	Minimum time	
T1	Man W/C car	IN	IN	IN	A	MA	Minimum time	
T2-T7	Man W/C car	IN	IN	IN	MA	IN	Minimum to none	
T8-T9	Man W/C car ?exercise ambulat.	IN	IN	IN	IN	IN	None	?KAFO
T10-T11	Man W/C car exercise ambulat.	IN	IN	IN	IN	IN	None	KAFO
T12-L1	Man W/C car ?house ambulat.	IN	IN	IN	IN	IN	None	KAFO
L2-L3	Man W/C car house ambulat.	IN	IN	IN	IN	IN	None	KAFO
L4 and below	Commun. ambulat. ?W/C, car	IN	IN	IN	IN	IN	None	AFO

*From Hussey R. W. (personal communication).
†D, dependent; IN, independent; A, needs assistance; MA, needs minor assistance.
‡KAFO, knee-ankle-foot orthosis; AFO, ankle-foot orthosis.

"mobility" (in bed, wheelchair, transfers in car, and driving) and dressing, grooming, and bowel and bladder care. Three categories of function were used: independent, semi-dependent, and dependent with the amount of human assistance as the criterion. If we use a 50% incidence of achievement in the population as the measure of what might be expected, those with C6 level were "independent" in wheelchair mobility only. They were "dependent" in bowel and bladder care and lower extremity dressing and required assistance in other areas. Those with C7 level (triceps intact as well as partial innervation of latissimus dorsi and sternal pectoralis muscles) had a considerably greater degree of "independence." They were generally able to function without any assistance in all areas aside from bladder care, lower extremity dressing, and driving.

It is important to recognize that "independent" function is not necessarily the goal of rehabilitation. The availability of caretakers may make it possible to choose to function in some areas with assistance rather than, for example, carrying out transfers alone using a sliding board. Thus, some of the tasks done "independently" at hospital discharge were being done on follow-up with assistance when this appeared to be more efficient. This illustrates that actual function reflects not only the level of neurological impairment but also the character of the environment, here the availability of a caretaker. The priorities in rehabilitation may thus differ.

In their assessment of the relationship between level of neurological impairment and ambulation, Hussey and Stauffer (5) found it useful to describe the actual remaining muscle actions rather than those that depend on the level of lesion alone. This was particularly true for those with an incomplete lesion or with injuries at the thoracolumbar junction, where a given skeletal injury can produce wide variations in actual function. Degrees of ambulation were defined: "community" ambulators were those able to walk for reasonable distances unassisted by another person; "household" ambulators were those who were able to walk within the home with reasonable assistance; "exercise" ambulators required controlled conditions and significant assistance in order to ambulate; and "nonambulatory" persons used the wheelchair entirely. The two highest categories reflected an effective level of mobility via ambulation that permitted the person to overcome physical barriers in the environment.

Motor power appeared to be the major but not the sole determinant of the level of ambulation achieved. Pelvic control was necessary in all instances. The quadriceps muscle seemed to be of paramount importance in determining the level of ambulatory function. Although 6% managed to achieve performance in the two highest categories without meeting that criterion, "fair" or better quadriceps function in at least one leg was generally necessary. The converse, however, was not necessarily true. Twenty-four percent of those at the exercise level and 10% of the nonambulators functioned at those lower levels despite adequate quadriceps function. Hip flexors also seemed to be contributing factor to effective function in most persons in the highest categories, but once again there were rare instances of persons in the two highest groups without such function. Hip abductors and extensors as well as knee flexors appeared to be less crucial. Although it was difficult to assess the effects of sensory findings per se, proprioception in the hips and knees also seemed necessary.

Community ambulation thus was likely given good pelvic control and active hip flexors and at least one quadriceps muscle in the fair or better range. Ambulation at the household level required pelvic control as an essential minimum with the presence of hip flexors necessary for most. The superimposition of age, deformity, or spasticity contributed to diminishing the functional level that the person might have achieved based on motor power alone. Those with motor function similar to that in community ambulators but affected by these or other superimposed conditions might be reduced to household ambulators. Thus, the examination of motor power alone does not entirely determine the level of function in real life.

Range of motion of an extremity and degree of resistance to passive stretching are two additional factors determining the actual function of the muscles. The assessment of the quantity and quality of resistance ("tone") can provide a basis both for improved function and for interference with function. For example, some persons with quadriparesis describe an ability to invoke a stiffening of the upper extremity that aids them in transfer. Persons with paraparesis can similarly evoke a stiffening of the legs in extension to aid in a standing transfer.

The motor portion of the neurological examination at times may require some modification in order to be more useful in the determination of the actual contribution to disabilities. For example, the MRC grading of motor power described in the previous chapter is particularly relevant to the function of the proximal joints, and the ability of the triceps to just extend the elbow against the weight of the forearm and the hand does signify useful function (grade 3). When applied to the ability to just flex a more distal joint such as a digit against its own rather little weight, this same criterion does not indicate the same degree of strength.

Moberg (2) thus suggests that the definition of useful function and thus the grade of "3" should not be in terms of movement against gravity for digits but some other criterion for a "weak but still useful muscle."

A further example of the evaluation of the upper extremity in relation to actual disability is the examination of the several shoulder muscles. These are important (along with the triceps) in raising one's body to relieve pressure on the buttocks and to manage transfer from bed to chair. The trapezius, pectorals, and latissimus dorsi are the muscles required. The combination of these several muscles can be usefully assessed by having the patient attempt to raise himself from his chair with his elbow in the examiner's hands. One may thus get an impression of the strength available for lifting the body as a combined action rather than as a function of individual muscles.

The assessment of strength in the latissimi is particularly difficult and may vary from that ordinarily expected on the basis of the already determined level of neurological impairment. Since the latissimi act to stabilize the back, their functional absence can be determined by observing that the patient chooses to hook his nonleading arm behind his wheelchair as a means of stabilizing himself. This use of the nonleading arm also indicates that this arm will be unavailable for any future development of a two-handed grip.

The assessment of certain specific muscles is particularly important in planning for the alleviation of disabilities by using them to replace actions that have been lost. The posterior part of the deltoid, for example, must be assessed separately, since surgical transfer may allow it to serve as an elbow extensor. In assessing the elbow flexors, it is important to separately examine strength in the brachioradialis, since it is frequently the only muscle that may be available for surgical transfer in order to achieve action at the wrist. Testing must be done with the elbow in 90° of flexion and the forearm pronated with the palm in the sagittal plane. One of the examiner's hands braces the forearm while the index finger of the other presses the muscle and tries to estimate its strength. It is important not to overestimate its strength if it is to take the role of wrist extensor after transfer. In general, transfer can be accomplished only if the muscle is rated at least 4/5 on the MRC scale prior to transfer.

Both the carpi radialis brevis and longus are responsible for extension of the wrist. This action can be the basis for hand grip when coupled with the passive movement of the fingers into flexion—the tenodesis hand. It is not possible clinically to differentiate the action of these two muscles, since the brevis—the more effective of the two—is innervated

TABLE 3-2. *Classification for Motor Function in Tetraplegia**

Group	Characteristics†
0	Weak BR and wrist extensors suitable together to provide wrist extension
1	BR
2	BR and ECRL
3	BR, ECRL, ECRB
4	BR, ECRL, ECRB, PT
5	BR, ECRL, ECRB, PT, FCR
6	BR, ECRL, ECRB, PT, FCR, finger extensors
7	BR, ECRL, ECRB, PT, FCR, finger and thumb extensors
8	Lacks only intrinsics

*From ref. 8.
† BR, brachioradialis; ECRL, extensor carpi radialis longus; ECRB, extensor carpi radialis brevis; PT, pronator teres; FCR, flexor carpi radialis.

from a part of the cord lower than the longus. It may thus be weak or paralyzed when the longus is functional. If the longus is used for transfer without first determining the availability of the brevis, wrist drop and a significant worsening of disability will occur. A technique has been developed to assess the action of the brevis with surgical exposure of the tendon. The movement of at least a 5-kg load is the criterion of its ability to work alone as a wrist extensor, thus freeing the longus for possible transfer to aid in other actions (1).

A number of classifications has been developed to describe the actual availability of specific muscles for actions of the upper extremities. Categorization on the basis of neurological level alone has proved too broad for functional planning, particularly when surgery has been contemplated (6,7). The internationally accepted classification, as described in Table 3-2, is concerned not only with the functionally significant muscles but with the availability of motors for possible transfer much later in life. It should be amplified by the availability of either cutaneous or ocular input.

Micturition

The relationship between impairments due to involvement of the sacral cord and to disturbances in bladder, bowel, and sexual functioning once again requires an analysis that goes beyond the usual clinical neurological examination. Table 3-3 describes a classification reflecting more precisely the effects of the neurological injury on both the urinary bladder detrusor and the sphincters (10) and attempts to reflect disabilities resulting from neurological impairment. The relationship between these

TABLE 3-3. *Classification of the Neurogenic Bladder**

1. Detrusor hyperreflexia
    Striated sphincter dyssynergia
    Smooth muscle sphincter dyssynergia
2. Detrusor areflexia
    Nonrelaxing smooth muscle sphincter
    Denervated striated sphincter
    Nonrelaxing striated sphincter

*From ref. 9.

categories and treatment procedures are described later (see "Bladder retraining").

The parasympathetic detrusor center arises from the intermediolateral cell column of S2-S4, with a major portion arising one segment higher than the more anterior pudendal nuclei innervating the striated urethral sphincter (11). The detrusor center innervates the body of the bladder, which is composed for the most part of cholinergic receptors and which contracts when acetylcholine is released. Conversely, the sympathetic outflow is inhibitory and promotes urine storage. Beta-adrenergic receptors in the bladder body lead to detrusor relaxation with epinephrine release. Conversely, the bladder base and proximal urethra contain more alpha-adrenergic receptors. Sympathetic stimulation produces smooth muscle contraction, described as the smooth muscle sphincter in Table 3-3. The sympathetic outflow arises from thoracolumbar segments T11-L1 (12).

Urine storage and micturition require a coordinated action of the bladder wall and the sphincter systems consisting of both striated and doubly innervated smooth muscles. Normally, an emptying contraction occurs when the bladder is full. The external (urethral) urinary sphincter, usually in a state of tonic contraction throughout filling, now relaxes. The emptying mechanism involves the detrusor smooth muscle, which is mainly but not entirely cholinergic. The contraction of the bladder opens the bladder neck, and urine passes out through the relaxed external urinary sphincter until the bladder is empty. The closing mechanism consists of the striated external sphincter of the urethra, other striated muscles of the pelvic floor, and the smooth muscle bundles of the bladder neck (mainly alpha-adrenergic). This normal alternating activity between the bladder detrusor and the sphincters has been called "reciprocation" and is under the control of the brainstem "micturition center" (13).

After the period of spinal shock, reorganization occurs within the disconnected cord. Those with lesions above the level of the sacral cord have an intact reflex arc of afferent input and motor output but without conscious perception. In most instances, the return of emptying on a reflex basis is possible, enabling as many as 70% of patients to become free of need for indwelling catheter. A major goal of the rehabilitation phase is to enable the person, particularly the male, to achieve a reflex bladder and thus avoid the need for an indwelling catheter. This is done in many instances at the cost of incontinence and the use of a condom catheter. The so-called upper motor neuron bladder has a greater likelihood of developing the pattern of detrusor hyperreflexia. Those with lesions at the level of the sacral cord and roots are more likely to develop the pattern of detrusor areflexia—the lower motor neuron bladder. These latter lesions may also display denervation of the external urinary sphincter but with more frequent retention of the internal sphincter innervation derived from the thoracolumbar system.

The findings on clinical neurological examination are helpful in distinguishing between these two major patterns but are not adequate for actual management. The presence of the bulbocavernous reflex and reflex contraction of the sphincter ani (anal wink) are consistent with the existence of the upper motor neuron pattern and the converse with the lower motor neuron pattern. In those with incomplete lesions, the finding on neurological examination of preservation of perianal sensation to pinprick was associated with the absence of symptoms involving the lower urinary tract. Impairment of such sensation was coincident with symptoms and/or abnormal findings on urodynamic studies. This correlation arises from the anatomical propinquity of the spinothalamic tract and the motor centers (11).

The ultimate, occasionally competing, goals of rehabilitation are to achieve and maintain low pressure within the bladder system to prevent ureteral reflux and hydronephrosis, limit the likelihood of urinary tract infection, and prevent incontinence. The particularly serious urological complications related to pressure within the system are delayed by catheter drainage, either urethral or suprapubic, but only delayed. There is therefore no easy way to achieve these goals. The longer-term management of the bladder cannot be predicted on the basis of neurological examination alone and requires urodynamic evaluation as well as visualization during fluoroscopy to determine the actual functional deficits that might interfere with achieving these goals.

It is useful to consider the problems to be either those of urine storage or emptying. Effective storage requires 1) the bladder to accommodate to increasing volumes of urine at a low intravesical pressure, 2) the bladder outlet to remain closed at rest and to remain so during intercurrent increases in intra-abdominal pressure, and 3) the absence of involuntary bladder contractions. Conversely, emptying requires 1) the coordinated contraction of an adequate magnitude of smooth muscle, 2) the lowering of resistance of the smooth sphincter, 3) lowering of resistance of the striated sphincter, and 4) no anatomical obstruction (12).

It would be convenient if the classification in Table 3-3 could be related directly to symptoms that the person with SCI could describe. However, a symptom such as incontinence can result from detrusor hyperreflexia and appropriately relaxing sphincters or from detrusor areflexia with sphincter denervation. Urinary retention due to neurological involvement may be due to detrusor hyperreflexia with sphincter dyssynergia or detrusor areflexia with either normal or nonrelaxing sphincters (14). It is necessary to determine the action of both aspects for proper management.

URODYNAMIC STUDIES

These include measurement in intravesicular pressure during filling, simultaneous measurement of intra-abdominal pressure (detrusor pressure being the difference), some measure of activity of the striated musculature of the pelvic floor by electromyography (EMG), and/or a measure of the pressure across the sphincters. Pharmacological intervention may also be carried out during course of observation. From the data generated, a number of determination can be made as to the character of the actual disability.

The degree of "compliance" of the bladder reflects the relationship of the change in pressure to the change in volume during filling. It is thus a measure of the accommodation provided by the bladder wall. In a normal bladder with a capacity of less than 500 ml, voiding occurs between 5 and 10 cm H_2O pressure. Compliance is said to be decreased if pressures are greater than 15 at filling.

No sudden increases in detrusor pressure should normally occur during filling; increased pressure should occur only with voluntarily initiated voiding. Sudden increases during bladder filling that cannot be consciously suppressed represent hyperreflexic contactility. Conversely, failure to develop voiding pressure leads to a classification of hyporeflexia. Bladder sensation is also assessed during filling as the "first desire to void." It is judged to be normal between 100 and 300 ml with diminished sensation when above the upper limits (11).

Lesions of the spinal cord above the sacral reflex arc disrupt the long tracts arising from the pontine centers responsible for coordination of the detrusor and the pudendal nuclei. There is not only detrusor hyperreflexia but also lack of coordination with the striated sphincter as measured by EMG. Unlike the normal cessation of sphincter activity during detrusor contraction, the activity may be either sustained or intermittent in relation to bladder contraction. Thus, "dyssynergia" is present. High sustained detrusor pressure can result in hydronephrosis. Excessive residual urine also generally occurs.

Residual urine has been used in the past as the criterion of a "balanced" bladder, with a residual of greater than 25% of the bladder capacity deemed significant. However, measurement of post-residual urine alone is insufficient to monitor the severity of the pressure. Some bladders develop severe hypertrophy (low compliance) with a predisposition to hydronephrosis and/or reflux without urethral obstruction due to dyssynergia. They will not show a high residual urine. Conversely, a high residual volume may be the result of inadequately sustained bladder contractions or inadequate relaxation of the internal bladder neck sphincter as well as the lack of external sphincter coordination (15). Thus, full urodynamic studies are necessary.

Bladder pressures below 80 cm H_2O are the maximum consistent with conservative management, but no absolute criterion can be used. The effects of intravesicular pressure leading to vesiculoureteral reflux and serious renal damage are the result of the duration high pressure has been maintained. Hence, high pressure prevailing with more frequent or prolonged contractions or during the relatively lengthy filling phase are particularly malignant (9).

Those with suprasacral lesions are further subdivided. Lesions above the level of the sympathetic outflow of the hypogastric nerve (T12) may display detrusor hyperreflexia with smooth muscle dyssynergia. There is a lack of coordination between the detrusor and the smooth muscle sphincter at the bladder neck, ordinarily innervated by alpha-adrenergic fibers. Associated dyssynergia of the external striated sphincter may or may not be present as well. The diagnosis of dyssynergia at the level of the smooth muscle sphincter is made on the basis of the effect of a short-acting alpha-adrenergic blocking agent (phentolamine) during urodynamic studies. A longer acting alpha-adrenergic blocking agent such as prazosin or phenoxybenzamine may then be indicated (16).

In addition to the disabilities in maintaining low intravesicular pressure and preventing infection and continence, those with lesions above T5 show the serious problem of massive sympathetic response to sometimes very slight degrees of bladder distension and contraction. Sweating, piloerection, headache, and hypertension are disproportionate responses when the supraspinal control of the sympathetic outflow is disconnected. The presence of this important syndrome of automatic dysreflexia is not limited to bladder distension, although such distension is the most common cause. This syndrome is discussed more fully later (see page 54).

Detrusor areflexia (lower motor neuron) occurs with lesions at the level of the detrusor nucleus (S2-S4) or the nerve roots, resulting in parasympathetic denervation. The absence of bladder contractions during filling would indicate detrusor areflexia. Bethanacol supersensitivity secondary to cholinergic denervation is determined by a rise in intravesical pressure of at least 20 cm of water above baseline with a bladder volume of 100 ml. In a group of patients with lesions of the conus and cauda equina (17), the bethanacol sensitivity test (BST) was found to be particularly sensitive for the presence of bladder denervation; it was positive in 95% of those with detrusor areflexia on filling.

EMG evidence of perineal floor neuropathy secondary to denervation includes giant polyphasic waves, fibrillation potentials, and positive sharp waves. Perineal floor neuropathy was evident in only 60% of those with a positive BST, illustrating the differing innervations of the detrusor and pudendal nuclei. Although the two are at the same level, the former is in the intermediolateral cell column, whereas the latter is in the ventral cell column. A variety of sphincter disturbances can thus co-exist with detrusor areflexia, as follows.

1. *Nonrelaxation of the smooth muscle sphincter.* Urodynamic assessment will show vesical areflexia with appropriate relaxation of the external urethral sphincter on EMG and improvement in flow rate or urethral pressure with alpha-adrenergic blockade. The maintenance of a closed bladder neck despite increased bladder pressure reflects continued sympathetic outflow with lesions below its exit from the cord at T11-L2. Animal studies also suggest that parasympathetic denervation increases alpha-adrenergic receptor activity in the urethral smooth muscle (14).

2. *A relaxed smooth muscle sphincter combined with detrusor areflexia and external sphincter denervation.* The bladder empties with only moderate increases in abdominal pressure and incontinence results. Urodynamic assessment will reveal vesical areflexia, and pudendal neuropathy will be indicated by EMG.

3. *Vesical areflexia on filling accompanied by continued or increased electrical activity from the external urethral sphincter as measured by EMG during attempted voiding with straining to increase intravesical pressure.* True dys-

synergia is not present, since there is no detrusor contraction, but rather a lack of relaxation of the urethral sphincter. Medications that affect skeletal muscle, such as those used for the treatment of spasticity, may be helpful.

These combinations illustrate the importance of not depending merely on the neurological examination and the determination of the existence of an upper or lower motor neuron pattern. Appropriate treatment can be determined only by also performing a complete urodynamic examination, which includes not only a cystometrogram but also EMG and urethral pressure measurements.

Defecation

The next perineal function to be considered early in the management of the person with SCI is bowel evacuation. The goal is to regain bowel control, i.e., to achieve regular and complete evacuation at a chosen time and place. This goal can be accomplished in the overwhelming majority of persons with SCI without the use of enemata and is generally far more easily accomplished than the adequate management of micturition.

Problems mentioned by patients include leakage of stool and the fact that bowel evacuation can take excessive periods of time on a daily or every-other-day basis, both of which interfere with the ability to function independently in the community. Incomplete evacuation at the chosen time and place is the major underlying problem, which can lead to the other disabilities. For example, the most common cause of loose stools is leakage around a site of fecal impaction. Abdominal discomfort due to distension is another consequence of incomplete evacuation. These problems may be present regardless of the level of injury, but their management will reflect the physiological consequences of the type of neurological impairment as well as the person's choice of lifestyle and bowel evacuation pattern prior to injury (18,19).

It is helpful to recognize analogies between micturition and defecation. The sigmoid colon is analogous to the urinary bladder as a site for storage. The rectum, normally empty except for the period immediately before defecation, remains closed by means of the continuous tonic activity of both a smooth muscle internal sphincter and the striated muscles of the sphincter ani and those of the pelvic floor such as the puborectal. Evacuation is a function of the contraction of the abdominal muscles to increase intra-abdominal pressure, the opening of the sphincters when sufficient stool enters the rectum, and the contraction of the rectal wall to expel the rectal contents.

The anatomical connections of the rectum are analogous to those of the bladder. A parasympathetic center in the intermediolateral cell column of S3-S5 causes contraction of the sigmoid and rectal muscles and relaxation of the internal sphincter, and the sympathetic system controls the reverse effects. Voluntary motor control courses in the lateral columns of the spinal cord, innervating the anterior horn cells of T6-T12 involved in the contraction of the abdominal muscles, and the sacral anterior horn cells that innervate the external sphincter and the other muscles of the pelvic floor (20).

On neurological examination, lesions above the sacral level are characterized by the contraction of the anal sphincter when the perianal skin is stimulated (anal wink), while lesions at the level of the conus and sacral roots are characterized by a patulous anus. Other relevant findings on examination would include the ability of those with low thoracic lesions to bear down using their remaining abdominal muscles to increase intra-abdominal pressure.

Normal voluntary control permits the subject to begin defecation, to withhold it regardless of the need to defecate, and to stop the activity in the middle or at the end. The mechanism for starting defecation is apparently the reflex act initiated by volition. Prolonged increased intra-abdominal pressure by bearing down relaxes the external sphincter. A more transient increase in intra-abdominal pressure is ordinarily compensated for by further contraction of the sphincter to guard against leakage.

Voluntary contraction of the sphincter also permits defecation to be withheld. It can be held contracted for up to 60 seconds, during which time the rectum automatically dilates to hold increasing contents at the same pressure. Rectal distension can cause this contraction of the anal sphincter even during sleep. Voluntary contraction of the anal sphincter and the pelvic floor muscles also provides the ability to stop defecation once it has begun.

Voluntary control of defecation is lost following complete transection of the spinal cord and interruption of the bilateral innervation of the sacral segments and defecation can be neither initiated nor stopped in the normal manner. Since no afferent impulses reach consciousness, there is no urge to defecate and no rectal pain. The person does not know when he is passing feces. Without an awareness of rectal events, the instinctive changes in intra-abdominal pressure that aid in defecation are lost, and it becomes more difficult to achieve complete evacuation at the appointed time and place. Stool may remain within the intestines, increasing the likelihood of fecal impaction as water is further removed, with possible subsequent leakage of liquid material around the blockage (21).

After the period of spinal shock, the intrinsic muscular activity of the bowel wall returns, and stool is moved through the colon to the rectosigmoid. The gastrocolic reflex is also apparently retained (22). Analogous to the urinary tract, the action of the lower portion of the bowel is most affected. However, even during the act of defecation, central pathways are not essential for the re-establishment of an efficient reciprocal relationship between the rectum and the sphincters.

The degree of disability and its management will vary with physiological pattern. For those with involvement above the level of S2, the anal sphincters are tonically innervated, the anus remains closed, and incontinence is less likely. With suprasacral involvement, rectal filling causes contraction of the external sphincter and a gradual relaxation of the rectal wall to accommodate its increased contents. As filling proceeds, the external sphincter becomes increasingly less able to contract, becoming fully relaxed and remaining so until evacuation has occurred. Automatic evacuation then occurs, as the terminal colon and rectum contract and both sets of sphincters are inhibited. As in the person with an intact spinal cord, evacuation is more likely if it occurs at an established time and in relation to the ingestion of food.

The volume of rectal contents required to initiate automatic evacuation has been found to be fairly constant, in the range of 100–150 ml. If the rectal wall has been chronically distended, the threshold needed to initiate evacuation is correspondingly raised. It is thus important to prevent stretching of the rectal wall during the course of bowel training. As with bladder distension, rectal distension may produce autonomic dysreflexia with hypertension and other evidence of an exaggerated sympathetic response in those with lesions above the level of splanchnic outflow (T5) (23).

Two other factors can contribute to controlled evacuation. As in the person prior to injury, an increase in intra-abdominal pressure such as by a cough or initial bearing down is at first excitatory of the pelvic floor muscles. If continued, the pelvic floor muscles and the external sphincter will relax, while the anus remains closed, signifying continuation of the tonic contraction of the smooth muscle internal sphincter. However, when distension of the anal canal occurs, as with digital stimulation, the same pattern of excitation is followed by relaxation. The anus becomes widely patent, proving that inhibition of both the internal and external sphincters has occurred, setting the stage for automatic evacuation at an appointed time and place.

With a lesion at the level of the conus or sacral roots, the lack of tonic contraction of the external sphincter makes incontinence more likely. There is generally an even greater reduction in the propulsive force of the rectal wall contraction, generally in the pressure range of 100–200 cm of H_2O. Those with a suprasacral lesion can develop a pressure of 60–100 cm, while the pressures available in those with a conus lesion are in the range of 40–60 cm of H_2O (4). The ability of the retained abdominal musculature to develop relatively high intra-abdominal pressures may contribute to the achievement of an appropriately timed evacuation. Unfortunately, concomitant problems in incontinence may occur at times of inadvertent bearing down when body movements normally occur. The ability of the sigmoid to act as a reservoir is unimpaired. One must thus aim to preserve the holding function of the colon; it is particularly important to ensure the complete emptying of both the sigmoid and the rectum at the appropriate time and place (19). The methods for dealing with these two major patterns of bowel movement are described later in this chapter (see "Bowel retraining").

Sexual function

The effects of SCI on sexual function are far more widespread than those affecting ability to carry out sexual acts involving the genitalia. Human sexual activity serves a complex need for personal expression and gratification, with numerous psychological, social, and aesthetic implications. The sex drive is not necessarily affected by SCI per se, but rather may be affected by pain or illness as concomitants of SCI, at least initially. The term "sexuality" is a broad term that encompasses the expression of sex drives through sexual acts in the context of the individual's identity—one's maleness or femaleness—and includes a range of behaviors from smiling through and beyond orgasm (25). Although all these aspects may be affected by the presence of SCI, this section focuses on the neurological background for disabilities relating to genital sexual activities.

The differential effects of the level of neurological impairment vary in a way similar to that of micturition and defecation in terms of the suprasacral (upper motor neuron) and sacral levels (lower motor neuron). Even more clearly than in other areas of impairment, the character of the disabilities and the functional consequences of the neurological injury reflect not only physiological aspects but the person in whom the injury has occurred and his or her life situation. The person's sex, age, and previously achieved level of sexual intimacy and the availability of a mate all contribute to making the character of the disability almost idiosyncratic to each individual. The significant disability for one may be the ability to achieve vaginal penetration but for another the ability to sire a child. Alternative means may be available that are then specific to each goal.

One aim of the initial rehabilitation in respect to sex might be to provide the person with information about the possible effects of SCI on sexual behavior. Also essential is an awareness that there are multiple options that have served others with SCI in meeting their needs for sexual intimacy. Individuals can then begin to assess their own goals and develop their own methods in terms of specific life situations.

For a woman, disabilities in sexual arousal and satisfaction may arise as a result of the loss of sensation in the perineal area. Fertility problems may arise in the management of contraception, since oral contraceptives may be contraindicated in light of the higher incidence of venous thrombosis in those with SCI, and the motor skills necessary for the proper insertion of a diaphragm may be lacking. Contraception, however, need not be affected, although pregnancy may make more troublesome an already compromised level of motor function. For those with lesions above the splanchnic outflow (T5), parturition may bring about autonomic dysreflexia.

For a man, disabilities may occur in erection and penetration as well as in the experience of sexual orgasm in relation to emission and ejaculation. Disabilities in fertility also occur, with problems of anterograde ejaculation as well as in producing an adequate number of viable sperm. The character of these disabilities differs somewhat with the level of neurological impairment.

Once again, analogies may be made to the innervation of the other perineal functions. Both cholinergic and adrenergic fibers as well as striated muscles are involved, with their complex interplay monitored and enhanced by sensory input. Erection of the penis (or clitoris) comes about by both tactile and cerebral stimuli, with sustained vasodilatation of the paired corpora cavernosa. Vasodilator adrenergic fibers from the sympathetic outflow (T12-L3) serve what has been called psychogenic arousal. Exteroceptive tactile stimuli as well as interoceptive stimuli from the bladder or rectum entering into the sacral cord lead to vasodilatation via the parasympathetic cholinergic fibers (S2-S4), termed reflexogenic erection. Although these two channels for achieving erection generally work synergistically, each may operate independently. For example, psychogenically induced stimuli may be inhibitory and hinder reflexogenic erections (26).

Emission involves movement of spermatozoa along the vas deferens, contraction of the seminal vesicles, and secretion by the prostate and accessory glands into the posterior urethra. In the plateau phase of male sexual arousal, the corpus spongiosum of the penis becomes engorged with blood with straightening of the urethral channel and the shaping proximally of a distended urethral bulb to hold the bolus of sperm and fluid. Animal studies confirmed in humans indicate that adrenergic stimuli from the lower thoracic and upper lumbar sympathetic ganglia are responsible for this first phase in the sequence of orgasmic experience. Reflex closure of the internal sphincter of the urinary bladder also occurs via adrenergic stimuli, preventing admixture of urine and sperm.

Ejaculation occurs by rhythmic contraction of the urethral bulb via stimuli from lumbar sympathetic nerves somewhat caudal to those described in relation to emission. Striated perineal musculature (ischiocavernosus and bulbocavernosus) is innervated by the pudendal nerve from sacral segments S2-S4. The contraction of these striated muscles propels the seminal bolus forward through the length of the urethra. Although orgasm is frequently thought to be synonymous with ejaculation, it should be considered a distinct event. The term orgasm refers to the subjective sensory feelings associated with ejaculation and emission, and may therefore potentially occur without the physical act of ejaculation (27).

According to Comarr (28–31), the clinical neurological examination of the relevant sacral segments consists of determining the presence or absence of reflexes such as the bulbocavernosus and anal wink, the ability to carry out voluntary closure of the anus, and the ability to respond to pinprick in the sacral region. If a patient has bilateral pinprick sensation in the penile, scrotal, and perianal areas, one may anticipate the return of psychogenic erections, ejaculation, and orgasm regardless of his ability to control the external anal sphincter. The categories of neurological impairments are reflexic (upper motor neuron) and areflexic (lower motor neuron), complete or incomplete within each category. This scheme of classification is based only on the examination of the somatic components of the sacral segments and not the crucial autonomic components of genital sex.

Based on Comarr's extensive experience, reasonably accurate predictions may be made as to the likelihood of disabilities in the various sexual functions in the presence of these different patterns. About 90% of males with "reflex complete" will have erections on a reflexogenic basis with tactile stimuli, and 70% of those will generally achieve succesful coitus. Most will not be able to ejaculate or have an orgasm during coitus, and psychogenic erections are almost unknown. The incidence of both erections and penetration increases for those who are "reflex incomplete"; 45% will have both psychogenic and reflexogenic erections, and approximately one-third of those who have successful coitus will also be able to ejaculate.

Most "areflexic complete" males do not have erections of any type. The relatively small percentage who do have them on a psychogenic basis. If their injury is below T12, at least some of the adrenergic fibers with supraspinal connections can reach the requisite organs. Success in coitus with those erections is less than for those whose erections are reflexogenic. About one-third of those who have successful coitus also ejaculate. Such ejaculations tend not to be forceful. For those who are "areflexic incomplete," the incidence of erections is quite high; 75% have erections successful for use in coitus, and about half are able to ejaculate and have orgasm.

In women, orgasm depends on the amount of sensation retained in the erogenous zones such as the nipples, clitoris, etc. Fantasy apparently plays more of a role in orgasm than in men. At least half the women in one series did not lose a single menstrual period, which makes early counseling concerning contraception choices necessary before the first home visit.

Male fertility ordinarily requires the anterograde ejaculation of a sufficient number of viable sperm. The actual siring of a child obviously depends on a large number of variables additional to the ability to ejaculate. However, in those relatively few persons with SCI who could ejaculate, the incidence of live births may approach 20%. Other methods of course exist to induce ejaculation, such as electrostimulation or vibratory stimulation. The earlier use of intrathecal prostigmine (32) to induce erection and ejaculation was discontinued after a person with a C6 lesion developed autonomic dysreflexia with cerebral hemorrhage and death. Artificial insemination after sperm collection by a variety of methods is possible.

The quality and number of sperm in those with SCI has long been felt to be a function of some modification of the neuroendocrine feedback loop. A defect in the negative feedback loop of the follicle-stimulating hormone (FSH), with increased basal levels of that hormone as well as a rise in the leutinizing hormone (LH), has recently been confirmed in persons with complete lesion below T12 (33). This correlates with testicular biopsy showing aspermatogenesis and loss of Sertoli cells, which are ordinarily responsive to FSH and LH produced by the pituitary. Circulating levels of testosterone were not significantly diminished in this small group of persons with SCI, although basal levels of these two pituitary hormones might serve as a signal of actual structural testicular defects of unknown pathophysiology.

In summary, erections are more probable in patients with upper level lesions, with the highest frequency in cervical lesions, while ejaculation is more frequent with lower level lesions. Successful coitus was highest in lumbar lesions, followed by cervical, upper thoracic, and lower thoracic. Tachycardia and hypertension may occur on ejaculation. For those with lesions above T5, the response will be exaggerated with autonomic dysreflexia (34).

Although these percentages help to assess the odds for various functions, they cannot, of course, predict the actual experience of any one person. There are exceptions to every rule. Only with time and attempts at coitus with a caring, responsive partner can one determine the limits of one's sexual activity.

Autonomic function

Impairments in the autonomic system produce disabilities that are frequently severe and, in several instances, unique to SCI (see Fig. 3-1). Effects on lower thoracolumbar sympathetic outflow and the sacral parasympathetic outflow were described in the context of bladder, bowel, and sexual functions. Impairments of the upper and midthoracic sympathetic outflow have major effects on total management. Vagal nerve activity is ongoing, since it arises from cell bodies above the foramen magnum. This has important functional consequences for temperature regulation and cardiovascular reflexes.

The *resting* pulse, blood pressure, and temperature may show no evidence of the underlying impairment; disabilities arise from impairments in the ability of the body to maintain homeostasis in response to changes in environmental temperature and change in position.

The neurons that eventually give off branches to the blood vessels of the abdominal viscera, muscles, and skin arise in the cell bodies of the intermediolateral cell column of T1-L4. Post-ganglionic alpha-adrenergic fibers stimulate active vasoconstriction in the vessels of the abdominal viscera and the skin. Post-ganglionic beta-adrenergic fibers cause vasodilatation of the vessels in the muscles in response to exercise and accelerate the heart. Sympathetic outflow to the large vascular bed of the intestines, carried by the splanchnic nerves arising from T5 T12, plays a particularly large role in the maintenance of blood pressure. Sympathetic outflow in the nerve supply of the skin are important for thermo-

REHABILITATION

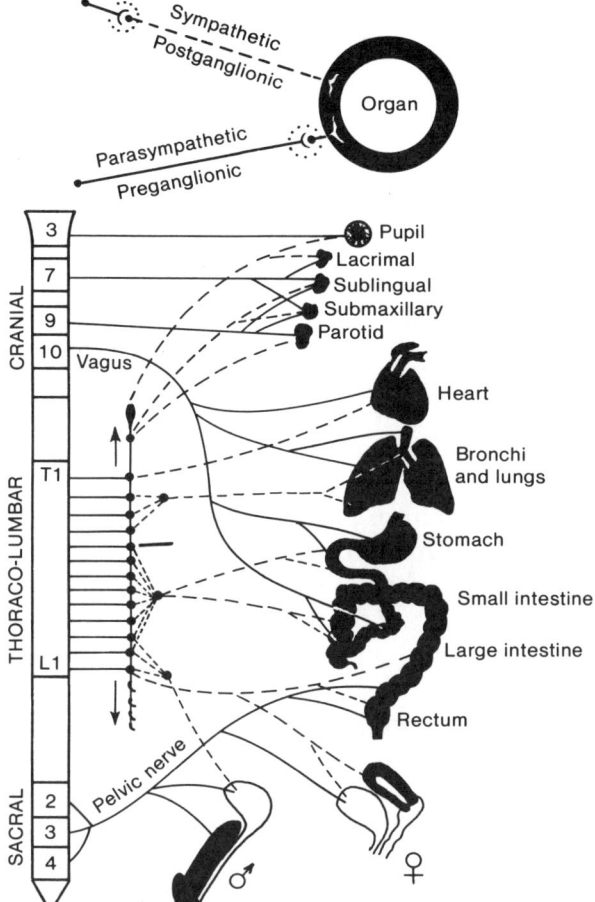

FIG. 3-1. The autonomic nervous system showing sites of origin within the spinal cord and organs innervated. The parasympathetic system has cranial and sacral origins, while the sympathetic system arises from segments T1 to L1. (Adapted by permission from ref. 20, 15th ed.)

regulation. In addition to their effect on blood vessels, post-ganglionic cholinergic fibers stimulate secretion of the sweat glands.

In the intact nervous system, the outflow to the muscles and skin represents two distinct mechanisms (35). Sympathetic activity in muscle is composed of impulse bursts discharged in response to the cardiac rhythm. Variations in afferent input from arterial baroreceptors lead to reciprocal changes in muscle sympathetic activity. The sympathetic innervation of the skin contains an admixture of sudomotor and vasoconstrictor impulses, which fire in bursts of varying duration and strength having no obvious relation to the cardiac rhythm. Skin sympathetic activity is influenced by arousal or emotional stimuli as well as by temperature.

THERMO-REGULATION

Afferent stimuli from temperature receptors on the periphery enter the spinal cord, ascend in the lateral spinothalamic tract, and eventually reach the hypothalamus. The anterior portion of the hypothalamus is apparently involved in heat loss mechanisms, the posterior portion with body warming. The efferent side of the reflex arc involves bilateral innervation of the sudomotor tract in the lateral area of the spinal cord. Fibers for the upper limb in this tract are more medial than those for the lower limb. After synapsing with cell bodies of the intermediolateral cell column, neurons exit through the anterior horn and innervate the skin via the chain of paired sympathetic ganglia.

Complete interruption of the sudomotor pathways between the hypothalamus and the sympathetic outflow abolishes the action of the sweat glands. The extent of the loss following a complete lesion depends on the level of injury and the time elapsed after injury. Initially, anhidrosis is more extensive and conforms to the level of sensory loss. With time, there may be a return of function several dermatomes below the original level.

In those with injuries above T1, there is initial anhidrosis over the entire body. With exposure to high temperatures, the only available compensatory mechanisms are panting and cutaneous vasodilatation. Sometime after injury, an improvement in vasomotor control and increased tolerance to heat occurs even in those with quadriplegia. With lesions below T4, the degree of supralesional hyperhidrosis increases with time, and additional sweating may occur well below the sensory level with continued exposure to high temperatures (36). However, unless the lesion is below T8, the skin surface capable of providing for heat loss through cutaneous vasodilatation and sweating is insufficient. For those injured above that level, air conditioning is usually recommended during the summers even in relatively temperate climates.

A loss of ability to elevate body temperature in the presence of cold was also found in those with lesions down to T4, since the limited amount of musculature above the level of lesion prevents the use of shivering to increase metabolism. Hypothermia then occurs with prolonged exposure. Those with lesions below T8 appear able to maintain body temperature with appropriate vasoconstriction of the skin as well as through shivering (36).

Those with quadriplegia or high thoracic lesions thus function as poikilothermics and have major problems with deviations from a neutral ambient temperature in the range of 27° C. These major disabilities remain, although they are somewhat attenuated with the passage of time following acute injury.

CARDIOVASCULAR REGULATION

The maintenance of mean arterial pressure in response to changes in position requires interaction of the vasomotor control of both peripheral arterial resistance and venous tone, which affects the return of blood to the central veins and the heart as well as the action of the heart itself. In the intact nervous system, stimuli reflecting changes in pressure measured by the baroreceptors at the carotid bifurcation (carried by the glossopharyngeal nerve) and receptors at the aortic arch (carried by the vagus) enter the vasomotor center in the medulla, which is also influenced by the hypothalamus.

Vasomotor fibers in the lateral columns of the spinal cord run a course somewhat different from sudomotor fibers. In a given case, vasomotility may be affected but not sweating, or vice versa. As in the sudomotor system, synapse occurs with cells in the intermediolateral column, with fibers then coursing out of the spinal cord through the anterior horn.

Fibers from the cervical sympathetic ganglia ascend from the upper thoracic level of the cord to innervate the heart. The effects on the heart of the adrenergic system are mediated through the $beta_2$ receptors. Responses to a fall in blood pressure include increasing conduction through the pacemaker and the atrioventricular node, decreasing the refractory period, and increasing intrinsic contractility. In response to a rise in blood pressure in the intact nervous system, slowing of the heart occurs due to intact vagal tone. Those with lesions at T5 or below have intact splanchnic nerve innervation, with the degree of such retention greater as one descends to T12. Those with lesions between T1 and T4 have intact only the adrenergic innervation to the heart. Those with cervical lesions lack all adrenergic outflow to the cardiovascular system but retain the vagal outflow.

The tilt table can be used to demonstrate difficulties in the maintenance of blood pressure. Those with lesions above T5 showed profound vascular maladaptation to change from the horizontal to the vertical as a result of the interruption of the splanchnic control. Rapid and uninhibited accumulation of blood in the abdomen and lower limbs occurs due to the loss of vasomotor control, particularly of the venous return.

Cardiac output cannot be maintained and syncope occurs. This is particularly found during the early stages post-injury. Regular and frequent change of position can be an important stimulus in setting up a vasoconstrictor response and restoration of control. An abdominal binder and/or oral ephedrine can help to compensate in the early stages of orthostatic hypotension until restoration is achieved, which can be anticipated even in those with quadriplegia (36).

The combination of all these effects can be illustrated by studies on a group of patients 3–6 months post-injury in whom both the orthostatic and exercise effects interacted (37). In those with low thoracic or lumbar lesions, blood pressure (BP) was maintained despite position and increased appropriately with exercise (ergometry). There was also a normal increase in heart rate (HR) to 150–170 during effort.

In high thoracic lesions, an increase in HR followed both orthostasis and exercise. When the patient was placed erect, the HR increased 20%, with further increase during ergometry. However, BP decreased in the erect position and was further decreased during effort. Apparently, vasodilation occurred in the muscles of the exercised extremity without compensatory vasoconstriction of the splanchnic bed.

Those with lesions of the cervical cord lacked the compensatory response in HR as well as BP with change in position. With effort, there was a slight rise in HR only to around 120, attributed to an inhibition of vagal tone.

In more chronic situations, studies (38) of persons with tetraplegia showed some increment in HR and impoved maintenance of BP both in relation to effort and change in position. The improvement in BP was attributed to alpha-adrenergic activity, since it was abolished by alpha blockers. The increase in HR was related to vagal tone or its inhibition, since it was abolished by atropine.

AUTONOMIC DYSREFLEXIA

The absence of supraspinal control of sweating and vascular tone is even more disabling in the syndrome of autonomic dysreflexia. The T5 cutoff point for the control of the splanchnic outflow once again is the significant level, above which exaggerated reflex sweating and hypertension occur. An increased response occurs to a variety of stimuli that ordinarily would produce a sympathetic response within the intact nervous system (hence the term dysreflexia), including change in position, nociceptive stimuli, or distension of a viscus. The anogenital area is especially susceptible, with distension or contraction of the bladder or bowel. Acute episodes can also occur during sexual intercourse and during parturition. More chronic episodes can be due to ingrown toenails and pressure ulcers as well as chronic bladder infection. Although both increased sweating and hypertension can occur, the pattern of response may vary from patient to patient and over time in the same patient (36). The uncontrolled rise in blood pressure can lead to possible intracranial hemorrhage and death.

Afferent impulses that normally elicit a sympathetic reflex, such as distension of a viscus, bring about arteriolar spasm in the vasculature of the skin and splanchnic bed, generating a rise in blood pressure. Baroreceptors in the carotid sinus and aortic arch then send signals to the vasomotor center, where efferent impulses to the heart lead to slowing via the vagus and, in the intact nervous system, vasodilation to compensate and maintain normal blood pressure. When the sympathetic system is disconnected from supraspinal control, the only available compensatory response is bradycardia. The rise in blood pressure and sweating continues unabated above the level of the lesion.

In the classic case described by Guttmann (36), a sharp rise in both systolic and diastolic blood pressure occurred coincident with contraction of a distended bladder. Skin temperatures below the level of the lesion fell markedly, indicating vasoconstriction, but rose above the level of the lesion. Venous engorgement above the level of the lesion includes stuffiness of the nasopharyngeal mucosa (Guttmann's sign). Pounding headache, either frontal or occipital, is the most serious complaint. Reflex sweating also occurs above the level of the lesion and may extend below. Cardiac output does not necessarily change, although arrhythmias appear on EKG along with the bradycardia.

The treatment of an acute episode of hypertension is a medical emergency unique to SCI. It is necessary to determine the probable cause, to relieve the distension of the bladder or bowel, and to reduce blood pressure by vasodilating medications, particularly alpha-adrenergic blockers. The use of local anesthetics prior to manipulation of the bowel or bladder can abort the afferent portion of the reflex arc. The severity of the symptoms will vary, with some persons reporting only sweating and headache. Awareness of the person's specific symptoms—flushing, a feeling of warmth, slowing of the heart, etc.—can also occasionally be useful in reducing the degree of disability. Such signals serve as a substitute for the normal sense of fullness of the bladder or bowel and therefore act as a signal for emptying on the part of the person with SCI.

The pathophysiology of the exaggerated autonomic response to nociceptive and other stimuli in persons with chronic SCI was recently explored via microelectrodes. Studies in both muscle and skin (35,39) delineated the character of the sympathetic outflow in isolated cord as measured by changes in skin resistance and vascular flow. Findings include a low level of spontaneous activity. Thus, spontaneous sympathetic activity in the intact nervous system appears to depend on supraspinal excitatory impulses. As in the uninjured, painful stimuli and those involving pressure in the bladder region were effective in causing sympathetic outflow. There was the expected disconnection between temperature and changes in sympathetic outflow to the skin, and loss of the relationship of cardiac rhythm and sympathetic outflow to the muscles. Although sympathetic activity increased over the low baseline, the rise was not greater than that found in normals. Thus, the explanation of the exaggerated hypertensive response on the basis of increased sympathetic activity in the decentralized spinal cord is not supported. Unlike the intact nervous system, vasoconstriction was prolonged when it did occur, and it functioned as a mass reflex with effects on both skin and muscle in parallel. Perhaps the crucial loss is that of supraspinal baroreflex control.

Minimizing Disabilities

The goal of the rehabilitation phase is to minimize the specific disabilities created by the neurological impairments. One enhances those abilities that remain by retraining and by the use of alternative methods, such as prostheses and technical aids of various sorts, to accomplish life activities. By the time the person with SCI has reached the rehabilitation phase, the contributions of medical and surgical treatments have become more limited. In addition to the retraining of specific skills, there is a more general training program that underlies all the others: to enable the person with SCI to learn to define his own concerns and goals and to participate in solving his own problems.

Bladder retraining

The proper management of bladder function is always disabling to persons with SCI and is the major problem in the continuing care phase. The goals of rehabilitation are 1) to achieve continence while preventing illness due to infection and stone formation, and 2) to achieve and maintain low pressure within the bladder system to prevent ureteral reflux and hydronephrosis. The process of bladder rehabilitation involves retraining the bladder and reeducating the person. Particularly in those with suprasacral lesions, the development of a reflex bladder appears to result from spontaneous reorganization of the nervous system below the level of the lesion. Nevertheless, there are important contributions by the person with SCI to the restoration of control. Recognition of this contribution by both the professional and the person with SCI is a major function in preparing the latter for his necessarily active role in the management of the bladder during the continuing care phase.

With the return of the bulbocavernosus reflex and the end of spinal shock, there is a variable time during which the bladder must continue to be protected against over-distension prior to the development of an "automatic" reflex bladder in those with suprasacral lesions. Some persons with suprasacral lesions do not develop the ability to "kick off." It is usually not possible to predict who will or will not be able to develop an automatic bladder.

Intermittent catheterization is done on a schedule appropriate to prevent the accumulation of more than 500 ml at the time of emptying. An output in the range of 2,000–3,000 ml/24 hours is generally sufficient to minimize infection due to stasis. These goals should be clearly recommended and agreed to by the person with SCI after explanation of their rationale. For those with lesions of the sacral outflow, this same management of intermittent catheterization would be continued indefinitely, depending on the action of the sphincter as described earlier.

The person with SCI should learn his or her signs of bladder fullness and possible prodromata of micturition. Although different from those prior to injury, and frequently idiosyncratic, they may be nevertheless consistent. Sweating, changes in temperature, increased spasticity, and an increase in heart rate are all symptoms that have served this purpose. Some palpate the area of the bladder to determine fullness. Once a sense of fullness occurs, the person can aid in initiating or completing micturition by selecting from a variety of alternative maneuvers. These include percussion over the bladder, or rubbing the skin over the pubis or on the inside of the thighs. Actual pressure on the abdominal wall (Crede maneuver) and/or bearing down or coughing are particularly helpful in those with a lower motor neuron bladder with an open sphincter.

It is also important for the person with SCI to determine the effects on his or her urine flow of such freely available drugs such as caffeine and alcohol. Those with quadriplegia are sensitive to position, with a markedly increased urine flow while lying flat. Each must develop an awareness of how to deal with his or her own idiosyncratic characteristics in terms of lifestyle. The intake of a rigidly prescribed amount of fluid per hour does not educate a person with SCI to meet the goals of bladder management in a real-life situation. For example, several newly injured young men doing well while in the hospital had markedly overdistended bladders when they returned to the hospital from their first evening out. They had drunk several bottles of beer but failed to understand the need to increase their catheterization frequency to compensate for the increased urinary flow.

It is important that the patient himself record the results of his catheterization in respect to the agreed-upon goals. Those with adequate hand function (generally C8 or below) not only record the results but carry out the catheterization. As reflex micturition begins to occur, males can begin to use a condom or other sort of external collecting device. The frequency of catheterization can be reduced as the amount of urine found on catheterization diminishes to the range of 100–200 ml. A rule of thumb is to divide the 24-hour catheterized volume by 500 to give the number of catheterizations needed. Generally the early morning catheterization is the last to go, although the actual pattern will vary with each individual.

The management of reflex micturition in the male often requires external sphincterotomy, and the resultant incontinence is then dealt with via an external collecting device. The criteria for success have included reduction in residual urines and, more specifically, decreased intravesicular pressure. Failures have resulted from poor detrusor contractility, bladder neck obstruction, or an incomplete muscle incision. Adverse effects on erectile capability may occur from this procedure. Bladder neck myotomy along with the external sphincterotomy is an additional alternative for those with smooth muscle dyssynergia (9).

Pharmacological treatment in conjunction with or instead of surgery can be understood in relation to the two basic functions—urine storage or bladder emptying. Urine storage is aided by anticholinergics to inhibit bladder contractility and/or drugs that increase outlet resistance, such as alpha-adrenergic agonists or beta antagonists. Facilitation of bladder emptying occurs mainly with decreased outlet resistance. This can occur at the level of the smooth muscle, using alpha-adrenergic antagonists or striated muscle with antispasticity drugs. The use of intravenous phentolamine in combination with pudendal nerve blocks during urodynamic studies can define the respective contributions of sympathetic and somatic innervation (40).

The achievement of a "balanced" bladder is the goal, as defined by regular emptying that occurs without high intravesicular pressure and with less than 100 ml of residual volume after voiding. If this is not achieved, there are several alternatives in the male to the use of an indwelling catheter on a long-term basis. Instead of developing adequate

REHABILITATION

emptying at low pressure at the price of sphincterotomy and resultant incontinence, long-term intermittent catheterization can be used in combination with anticholinergic medications to paralyze detrusor function. This procedure has become increasingly accepted as an effective significant alternative in the management of a low intravesicular pressure system. An external collecting device can also be used to ensure dryness. This alternative requires training the person with SCI to adjust his or her fluid intake and the timing of catheterization to meet the flexible needs of community living.

The absence of an effective external collecting device in females makes it necessary to continue long-term intermittent catheterization with paralysis of detrusor function. A waterproof undergarment may be worn between catheterizations to avoid embarrassment. The difficulties of this regimen cause many women to choose constant indwelling catheter drainage despite its drawbacks.

Although urodynamic studies are frequently indicated for the ultimate management of the bladder, they should be reserved for those who are not making good progress after 9–12 months. Autonomic dysreflexia, recurrent sepsis, or continued high post-voiding residuals indicate a need for earlier study preparatory to a surgical procedure such as sphincterotomy (10) or more adequate pharmacological management (41).

Bowel retraining

Evacuation can be brought under control in the overwhelming majority of cases of SCI; emenata and cathartics are rarely necessary. The goals to be achieved are 1) continence, 2) the prevention of illness and discomfort due to inadequate elimination, and 3) the accomplishment of these goals without requiring an inordinate amount of time for bowel care. Just as with the bladder, the development of reflex bowel evacuation in suprasacral lesions appears to result from spontaneous reorganization of the nervous system. Nevertheless, there are important contributions that the person with SCI can make to achieving control, particularly those with lesions in the area of the sacral outflow, where incontinence is more likely. Such participation is an essential part of the process of learning to manage this crucial aspect of life in the continuing care phase.

Regular and complete evacuation at the appointed time and place requires management to prevent stool from remaining too long in the gut, since water absorption then results in impaction followed by diarrhea around the area of blockage. As with bladder function, some persons can identify some consistent signal of rectal distension, albeit different from that used prior to injury. Early signals of autonomic dysreflexia such as sweating or an increase in spasticity are some of the signals used. However, as with bowel training in childhood, it is particularly useful to establish a fixed time for evacuation. Just as before the injury, it might be useful to establish a time in relation to meals or the use of coffee. As with bladder retraining, it is important that a regimen of bowel evacuation be established early, to avoid overdistension of the rectal wall. Once a pattern has been re-established with stimulatory suppositories, it is generally possible to reduce their use and to depend solely on dilatation of the anal sphincter, either digitally or by a glycerine suppository. Those with lesions of the sacral outflow may not be able to develop enough intra-abdominal pressure to achieve evacuation and may require actual manual evacuation. The frequency with which one evacuates the bowels will differ, but several times a week is sufficient in most instances.

The person with SCI must understand the mechanisms by which bowel contents may have a relatively short transit time, to prevent bowel impaction without causing loose stools. Exercise is helpful, as it is in those with an intact spinal cord. Adequate fluid intake is necessary if dietary fiber is to be effectively used. The amount of fiber and its sources cannot be predetermined. Each person with SCI should select the amount and sources depending on his or her own preferences and the results achieved. Many will identify particular foods that cause them to have an almost immediate bowel evacuation. Although most people find it desirable to forgo such foods, some find it helpful to use them deliberately when they wish to empty their bowels. Table 3-4 lists some sources of dietary fiber that could be used by patients to design their own diet.

Sexual reintegration

The expression of one's sexuality after recovery from the acute effects of SCI requires in many instances a reorganization of one's sense of self. Sexual reintegration includes the development of ways to deal with the implications of impairments, not only in the specific act of carrying out sex but in terms of one's entire physical appearance. In addition, sex is a social encounter rather than just a physical one. The term sexuality encompasses how one expresses the social role of a male or female in any particular culture (25).

Reintegration is thus a complex process that goes beyond focusing on the mechanics of sexual union. No outside guidance can possibly de-

TABLE 3-4. Fiber Content of Food*, †

Food	Amount	Grams of dietary fiber
Breads and cereals		
All-Bran	⅔ cup	17.0
Bran Buds	⅔ cup	15.8
Bran Flakes	¾ cup	4.0
Corn Flakes	1 cup	0.5
Grape Nuts	½ cup	2.8
Oatmeal	¾ cup	1.6
Puffed Wheat	1 cup	0.5
Rice Krispies	1 cup	0.1
Shredded Wheat	1 biscuit	2.2
Special K	⅔ cup	0.1
Whole wheat bread	1 slice	2.1
White bread	1 slice	0.7
Bran muffin	1 medium	3.5
Fruits		
Apple, raw with skin	1 medium	2.8
Applesauce	½ cup	1.4
Apricots, raw	3 medium	1.4
Apricots, canned	6 halves	0.8
Banana, raw	1 medium	1.6
Blackberries, raw	½ cup	3.3
Cantaloupe, raw	1 cup	0.5
Grapefruit, raw	½	0.5
Orange	1 medium	2.8
Peach, raw	1 medium	0.5
Peach, canned	½ cup	0.5
Pear, raw	1 medium	4.1
Pear, canned	½ cup	1.2
Pineapple, canned	½ cup	0.9
Prunes, dried	4	5.4
Strawberries, raw	1 cup	2.8
Vegetables		
Asparagus	½ cup	1.5
Avocado, raw	½ medium	2.3
Beans, green	½ cup	2.0
Broccoli, cooked	⅔ cup	4.1
Brussels sprouts, cooked	6–8 medium	2.9
Cabbage, raw	½ cup	1.7
Carrots, raw	1 large	2.9
Carrots, cooked	⅔ cup	3.1
Cauliflower, raw	½ cup	1.0
Cauliflower, cooked	½ cup	1.1
Celery, raw	2 stalks	1.8
Corn on cob	4-inch ear	4.7
Cucumbers	1 medium	0.4
Lettuce	3½ ounces	1.5
Mushrooms	10 small	2.5

(continued)

TABLE 3-4. *Fiber Content of Food (cont'd)*

Food	Amount	Grams of dietary fiber
Peas, green, canned	⅔ cup	6.3
Peppers, green	¼ large	0.2
Potatoes, mashed	½ cup	0.9
Potato, baked	1 medium	2.5
Spinach, cooked	½ cup	6.3
Tomato, raw	1 small	1.5
Tomato, canned	2/5 cup	0.9
Other		
Graham crackers	4 squares	0.8
Ryekrisp	2 triple crackers	1.6
Wheat snacks	15	1.1

*From ref. 42.
† Fiber may be measured as either crude fiber or dietary fiber. This chart lists values for dietary fiber of some common foods.
Cup = 8-ounce measure.

termine the method by which any particular person will reorganize himself or herself in respect to this important area of human function. The rehabilitation process must be flexible in responding to the varieties of degree of neurological impairments coupled with the individuality of the ways people interact in human relationships. This section therefore attempts to establish principles rather than detailed approaches.

The treatment of disabilities related to sexual function illustrates to a particular degree what should be the overall goal of any rehabilitation program. It must serve to develop within the person (and partner) an ability to monitor one's own signals, to communicate one's own needs, and to continue to learn to solve problems as they arise. It is important for the person with SCI to learn in this context to become clearer about his goals or the outcomes sought, and to differentiate between outcomes and the means or actions by which one may go about achieving them. Just as with those who are able-bodied, goals will vary. For one person, the important goals might relate to the siring or bearing of children while, for another, the priorities are to be physically intimate with another person, or to achieve pleasure, or for still another to dominate.

One young man with paraplegia for the previous five years found it helpful to consider what he was seeking in a sexual relationship. For him, the goal was to reach a level of excitement and pleasure similar to that he had looked for before his injury. When he became clear about

REHABILITATION

what he wanted, the means or methods fell into place for him. "What was 'normal' for me was to do whatever I needed to meet my goal. The goal was the same as before even if I did do some things differently."

Another man with long-standing quadriplegia found, when he asked himself the same question, that his thinking was different from what it had been when he was both younger and uninjured. Now in his second and more emotionally satisfying marriage, he feels that he is looking for a deeper sense of sharing with his mate. His sexual relationship brings him intimacy with another person and a sense of physical release, albeit qualitatively different from before. Although he did not ejaculate or have the same sort of orgasm as in the past, he was satisfied with what he did experience, which he called "mental orgasm."

In addition to defining relatively clear goals, it is necessary to develop a sense of options, of alternative means by which one can achieve these goals. A number of sources of information for such alternatives are available, most usefully other persons with similar disabilities (42). What others have done is not as helpful as the awareness of the range of alternatives that other people have used. The professional must respect the right of the person with SCI and his partner to select those options that are appropriate for them.

The means by which an individual may be aroused can differ from that prior to injury. Masters (personal communication) describes a woman who had been studied before and after injury. Her breasts had not been before, but became after injury, a major site for sexual stimulation, replacing those sites that were below the level of her lesion. Similarly, he describes the ability to experience flushing and other sympathetic nervous system effects above the level of lesion, compatible with those experienced prior to injury in the pelvic region during orgasm.

The principles of treatment for persons with SCI are similar to the treatment of sexual disabilities in the general population. Drugs such as anticholinergics that might interfere with function should be reviewed. Although impotence may be based on neurological impairment, performance anxiety can be superimposed. Counseling of both partners before their getting together can help prevent the initial failure that can establish a future pattern of failure (43). Counseling might usefully include such concepts as: the absence of sensation does not mean the absence of feelings, the inability to move does not mean an inability to please, an inability to perform does not mean an inability to enjoy.

A number of medical and surgical methods are available to supplement the degree of erection. Externally applied vacuum-type pumps increase blood flow, which is then held within the penis by a tourniquet arrangement (44). The surgical insertion of semi-rigid rods or inflatable bags within the corpora cavernosa have helped many men with SCI to achieve effective erection, despite a relatively high incidence of infection (45). These rods have also been useful in enabling men to use condoms for urine collection when their phallus was not ordinarily adequate for them to do so. More recently, there has been a resurgence of interest in the use of nonhormonal pharmacological treatment (46). In selected cases, papaverine combined with alpha-adrenergic blockers such as phentolamine have been used to simulate the increased arterial flow and relaxation of smooth muscle walls within the corpora cavernosa that occur with natural sexual arousal.

Skin management

Prevention of pressure sores in the newly injured person primarily depends on the staff carrying out a 2–4-hour turning schedule. With the end of spinal shock, there is a gradual improvement in vasomotor tone, and some reduction in this frequency is generally possible. Vasomotor tone does not appear to remain the major factor in the incidence of pressure sores. Overall, there is a greater frequency of sores in those with paraplegia than in those with quadriplegia despite continuing problems with vasomotor control in the latter.

Education in skin management during rehabilitation provides an important opportunity for preventing later morbidity and even mortality. Information on the prevention of burns due to exposure to heat, the prevention of cuts by avoiding sharp objects, and keeping the skin clear of urine and feces are all obviously appropriate. The major unique focus in persons with SCI is the need to prevent skin breakdown due to prolonged pressure, in the absence of the usual sensory input.

Beginning to sit in a wheelchair and entry into motor training programs lead to an increase in the opportunities for skin breakdown. The goal remains prevention of skin breakdown, but the means now depend to a far greater degree on the person with SCI.

Ischemia of the skin and the underlying tissues occurs particularly in weight-bearing areas adjacent to bony prominences. For example, "sitting" sores are most frequently associated with the ischial tuberosities. Pressure directly over these bony protuberances can exceed 300 mm Hg on an unpadded seat, and are decreased only to 150 mm Hg by 2 inches of foam padding. Even with the use of cushions designed to distribute pressure, the pressures in the sitting position are far above those in the capillaries or venules (11–33 mm Hg). The period of time over which pressure is applied to a tissue is the most significant variable relating to the maintenance of integrity. Even relatively low pressures over a long period of time can cause necrosis unless a sufficient "rest period" is given (47). Consistently maintained pressure above 33 mm Hg effectively blocks venous return and the removal of metabolic waste, leading to edema and eventual focal injury (48).

Pressure is also concentrated in deeper tissues that are closer to the bone, and fat and muscle resist pressure less well than does skin. These factors contribute to the occasional finding of a small cutaneous ulcer overlying a much larger area of fat and muscle destruction. Still another factor is the importance of parallel as well as perpendicular forces. Raising the head of the bed by only a few inches may increase the shearing force over the sacrum high enough to deprive large areas of their necessary blood supply. Very large ulcers can be produced by friction when the patient is slid down the bed. In animals, ulcers can be produced with far less perpendicular pressure when shear or parallel movement is added.

It is particularly advantageous to learn of possible ischemia. Even those with complete lesions describe a sense of burning in the buttocks or some other relatively poorly localized signal related to sitting for long periods. A change in the pattern and amount of spasticity is another common signal. Pressure relief precludes skin breakdown by preventing the appearance of such signals of ischemia. Methods for pressure relief vary considerably, with lift-offs by those with paraplegia and some other means of weight adjustment by those with quadriplegia. In the absence of signals arising from the body itself, many schedule pressure relief every 10–15 minutes. The frequency of pressure relief and the total time spent sitting each day cannot be arbitrarily prescribed. Each person must develop an appropriate program based on variations in his general state of health, the toughness of skin, and many other factors. Scars from previous episodes of skin breakdown are particularly susceptible.

The success of one cushion over another to distribute pressure more equally cannot be predetermined. One person with quadriplegia described his success in preventing skin breakdown by monitoring the appearance of his skin over many years. When he noted erythema after sitting the usual time duration and with his usual methods of pressure relief, he would look for another cushion that might work better. In testing the several different systems (gel, foam, air, and so forth), he found that a widely recommended one caused him to sweat excessively and thus produced erythema of the buttocks. By sampling several systems, he found one that provided him with the best results.

In addition to diffusion of pressure, other criteria for wheelchair cushions include heat dissipation and weight. Gels, for example, help inhibit rises in skin temperature due to their high heat capacity as compared to polyurethane foam but fail to reduce interface moisture, since there is no opportunity for the air exchange available in foams. A layered combination of materials has been suggested to take advantage of the characteristics of the several materials available for design appropriate for different individual's weights and other needs (49).

After the prevention of skin ischemia, the next set of goals is for the person with SCI to learn to identify early signs of incipient skin breakdown. The specific findings will vary with the pigmentation of the skin. Rubor or other change in color, induration, and blistering are several signs that occur prior to actual break in the skin. A mirror and skin palpation should be used by the person with SCI or a caretaker on arising and after sitting, with particular attention paid to bony prominences such as the ischia, trochanters, and sacrum as well as sites of previous scars.

Once such signs are found, a way must be established to prevent further injury and permit healing. The sine qua non of any program must be pressure relief. One person with quadriplegia described how the appearance of a "pimple" on his sacrum was a signal for him to avoid all sitting for several days so that healing could occur. Surgical removal of a chip of bone in the sacral region eventually reduced his likelihood of ischemia. However, because of this careful management, actual breakdown of the skin did not occur.

The program for pressure relief in the presence of a signal of incipient breakdown varies with the individual's way of living and the availability of caretakers. The aim is to achieve as complete pressure relief as possible. It is frequently possible even for those living alone to reduce the amount of sitting time necessary to carry out daily activities. Early sores that involve the epidermis or dermis only (Grades 1 and 2) may be managed by pressure relief alone. Fat necrosis and the appearance of muscle in the wound (Grade 3) may require debridement (47). Grade 4 describes involvement of bone or joint, which requires long-term hospitalization. One objective in a skin management program has been to monitor early wounds closely and to provide more thorough pressure relief in the hospital for those who are not improving. With early referral, one can prevent the need for more costly and extensive surgical treatment, which includes skin grafts and flaps to cover deep wounds.

If deep wounds occur, treatment again depends mainly on pressure relief by alternating weight-bearing surfaces. Although special mattresses and padding may make nursing care technically easier, it is clearly possible to heal pressure ulcers without them. Multiple wound sites that prevent effective alternation of weight-bearing necessitate air-fluidized mattresses. All the basic principles of wound care remain applicable, including removal of necrotic tissue, treatment of wound infection, and adequate drainage.

Although much can be accomplished by medical and surgical treatment of skin wounds, the major focus must be on prevention. In the absence of prevention of ischemia, early identification becomes the goal. In the absence of early identification and adequate self-help pressure relief, early referral then becomes the goal. At every stage, it is essential that the person with SCI participate in specifying the goal and the means for its accomplishment, since he must assume the major responsibility for carrying it out.

Mobility retraining

Traditionally, a major focus of disability in those with SCI has been mobility, since the loss of motor strength in the legs and consequent loss of ambulation has been one of its most salient features. Although standing may be quite valuable in its own right, this section is limited to methods for achieving functional mobility both in the household and in the larger community. The selection of techniques must eventually dovetail into other community resources such as mass transit, automobiles, or vans. The process of identifying the components of this community system depends on the previous exploration with the user of his life pattern and the physical environment. For example, one must be specific about such aspects as whether the person goes to restaurants, has been athletic, and is or is not comfortable in dealing with technology, as well as his home and work setting.

Safety is a paramount goal in achieving ambulation as a major component of mobility. Braces can substitute for weak muscles and create a stable basis for support. The more generic term "orthosis" is used to describe "an externally applied device that modifies structural and functional characteristics of the musculoskeletal system" (50). Functional electrical stimulation (FES) represents a means of achieving "active orthosis" as opposed to the more passive support of braces. The limiting factor in ambulation with the use of braces, crutches, or FES is energy expenditure and efficiency of time.

One result of the recent research interest in FES is new insight as to the contribution of various muscles to efficient function in standing and bipedal gait. The actual contribution of specific muscles to ambulation requires their analysis in relation to the gait cycle, defined from the heel strike of one foot to subsequent heel strike of the same foot. The cycle is subdivided into the stance and swing phases; the stance phase (60%) is the time that the foot is touching the ground, and the swing phase (40%) is that time the foot is off the ground swinging through to the next heel strike. During this period, the opposite foot is in the stance phase.

The hip extensors and hamstrings stabilize the hip and knee during the stance phase. The quadriceps muscle group is the major factor controlling the degree of stability at the knee, and bilateral FES of the quadriceps alone is sufficient to maintain standing (51). The hip joint is hyperextended, with balance and stability maintained by the arms and a walker or parallel bars. Switching FES to various muscle groups simulates the intermittent character of postural control and increases the time that standing can be maintained. Once the quadriceps has been stimulated, subsequent FES of the gastrocnemius and soleus group will maintain the posture while simultaneously diminishing the contraction of the quadriceps (52).

The dorsiflexors of the foot let it down gradually during the start of the stance phase and provide for pickup of the toe during the swing phase to prevent the foot from dragging or causing the person to stumble. An early use of FES was stimulation of the peroneal nerve in the knee region to correct footdrop in persons with hemiplegia (53).

The production of FES-assisted bipedal gait has presented a number of serious problems (51). Candidates have been persons with mid- to low thoracic level spinal cord injuries with muscular response available to electrical stimulation (upper motor neuron). Although some success has occurred in highly selected persons with SCI, major problems exist in the amount of energy required as well as the sensory inputs necessary, in addition to vision and hearing, to make the system more adaptive.

Following stimulation of the quadriceps to bring about stance, external stimulation in the peroneal region to elicit the accentuated flexor withdrawal reflex present in SCI is one method for bringing about flexion of the leg for the swing phase. Unfortunately, these responses have been inconsistent (54). Another method has included stimulation via implanted electrodes of muscles for both the support and swing phases (55). The quadriceps was utilized for knee extension, the iliopsoas for hip flexion, the posterior aspect of the adductor magnus for hip extension, and the soleus for plantar flexion. For those whose iliopsoas was not effective for hip flexion, the tensor fascia lata and sartorius were implanted. The anterior portion of the adductor magnus was then implanted to balance the external rotation and the abduction produced by the sartorius and the tensor, respectively. One finding in such studies has been a revision of the understanding of the action of muscles such as the adductors. The adductor magnus, for example, produced either flexion or extension depending on the position of the hip.

In those with intact hip flexors and proprioception at the hip, a knee–ankle–foot orthosis (KAFO) can provide knee stability when combined with forearm crutches to compensate for absent hip abductors. Knees are locked into neutral or a slight degree of flexion and the ankle joints are locked into slight dorsiflexion (10°). The swing-through gait that can be achieved permits mainly household ambulation. Persons ambulating with braces and crutches use from five to eight times as much energy as able-bodied walkers. There is some variation in efficiency depending on the type of orthosis, with the Scott-Craig brace somewhat more efficient (56). A manual wheelchair is usually used outside the home.

The training program for bilateral KAFOs involves upper extremity and trunk strengthening and endurance training, and hip flexion contractures must be reduced. Range of motion of the hamstrings with knees extended must be 110° in order for the person to don orthoses and come to standing from the wheelchair or from the ground [see Peterson (57) for a fuller description].

Those with normal proprioception at the knee and preserved knee extension against resistance but dorsiflexor weakness can use an ankle–foot orthosis (AFO). When the ankle dorsiflexors are weak and proprioception is absent, the ankle must be locked in the range of 5–10° of dorsiflexion. Persons able to function with bilateral AFOs can achieve mobility with an energy expenditure calculated as three to four times normal, which permits considerably more ambulation at a "community" level than do KAFOs (58). Once again, a manual chair is used for long distances. It is particularly crucial for these persons to learn to check for skin breakdown on the heel, in the absence of sensation on this weight-bearing surface. Peterson (57) has described the criteria for working with those with cauda equina lesions and varying degrees of proprioception, as well as variation in the strength of the muscles controlling the foot.

The overwhelming majority of individuals without knee extension on at least one side will use a wheelchair as their primary means of mobility (5). The design of the appropriate wheelchair is a function not only of the individual's level of neurological function and physical dimensions but also of his goals in life and the character of the environment in which he is to function (47). One man with SCI emphasized, "the wheelchair is not just a mode of transportation but an extension of one's body, enabling the person to participate in everyday living." One may consider the wheelchair analogous to a prosthesis in that it is "an artificial substitute for a missing body part." Like any other prosthesis, it is an extension of the body, to which it must fit while enabling the user to interact more effectively with a sometimes hostile environment.

Most persons with a functional level of C6 or lower will use a manual chair. Some whose level is C5 can be mobile in a manual chair adapted with push rims having projected pegs or plastic coating to increase grip. The need to travel long distances rapidly at work or school may make a power chair more practical when upper extremity function is impaired.

Persons with injuries at the C5 level or above require a powered chair. A powered reclining back is indicated to permit pressure relief on a regular basis for those without at least "fair plus" elbow flexion (59). Most can use a proportional hand controller, but a nonproportional controller is safer if spasticity is marked. A chin control can be used if only head and neck movement is available. If head and neck control is not present, breath control is an option. A manual chair should always be ordered as a backup to the power chair to be used while the latter is being repaired.

Given these general constraints, which depend on the level of injury, the actual degree of performance and mobility that may be achieved has improved with more recent modifications to the chairs. The introduction of lighter-weight chairs has enabled the user to re-enter society more easily. The reduction in weight makes it possible for the marginal user to fold his own chair, place it in his car, make it up a hill he could not climb before, maneuver more easily in tight places such as restaurants and stores, and even travel more freely with others, who need lift only 30 rather than 50 lbs.

The actual process of fitting the wheelchair to the person is undergoing even more fundamental changes, as the "generic" wheelchair to which the user had to fit is no longer the only choice. "Modular" wheelchairs permit a far greater variety of alternatives in response to the person's measurements, and some models also permit adaptation in response to changing needs.

Seat width should be the narrowest possible in order to achieve the narrowest frame width, to optimize clearance of doorways and other environmental barriers. The generic 18-inch or narrower 16-inch seat width can be adjusted even more precisely to the person's actual hip-to-hip dimensions with adequate clearance from the wheels. Seat depth should distribute weight along the buttocks and upper legs. Measurement from the most posterior portion of the buttocks to the back of the knee should subtract 2–3 inches to allow adequate clearance between the front of the sling seat and the back of the knees. Footrest length is measured from the back of the knee to the bottom of the heel with the knees slightly lower than the hips. Frame length should be such that the heel of the foot falls forward of the bend of the knee. Armrests are similarly adjusted to height.

Backrest measurement is taken from the posterior buttocks to the scapula. As a general rule, the backrest for a paraplegic should fall just below the inferior angle of the scapula and just above that angle for a quadriplegic. Those who participate in wheelchair sports can increase maneuverability by lowering backrests. Training in trunk balance can enable others to trade off a lowered backrest in return for a similar increase in maneuverability.

Brubaker (60) recently emphasized the options for increased mobility and performance based on the distribution of weight relative to the axis of the main wheels. He points out that rolling resistance is decreased, side slope effects minimized, and propulsion efficiency increased by placing the large rear wheels closer to the center of gravity. The ability to control the chair in a "wheelie" position, thus increasing maneuverability and curb climbing, is similarly enhanced by decreasing the distance between the center of mass and the axis of the wheels. In contrast, the "generic" chair sought static stability to prevent pitching forward by lengthening the horizontal distance between the body and the rear wheels. On the vertical axis, the generic chair raised the distance between the body and the rear wheels to ease transfer while simultaneously diminishing performance.

Such tradeoffs can thus be determined in respect to the goals of the person, his physical characteristics, and the demands of the environment. Moving the large rear wheels forward, closer to the center of gravity, provides a tighter turning radius that is helpful in indoor settings and a stronger stroke, while simultaneously increasing the likelihood of tipping forward. Moving the wheels rearward increases static stability and the ability to track for longer distances, which would be appropriate outdoors. Moving the wheels higher in relation to the seat also increases the strength of the stroke, by moving the wheels closer to the arms, but simultaneously raising the wheel relative to the buttocks makes transfer more problematical for some. In a similar fashion, the height of the seat relative to the wheels can vary for persons particularly interested in reaching high or reaching low, and for those situations when the height of tables and desks becomes more or less significant.

It is important to define the specific criteria to be established with the input of the person who will use the wheelchair. For some, variability in their needs makes it desirable to use a wheelchair that permits the user to adjust the relative position of the rear wheel axle to the seat in both the horizontal and vertical planes. To the extent that the user is able to modify these components, the wheelchair more nearly fits his individual circumstances and changing needs, even on a daily basis. The opportunity for change over somewhat longer intervals is particularly helpful to the newly injured, whose capabilities and expectations may increase with time.

The seating system contributes to the proper use of the wheelchair. In addition to the issues of diffusion of pressure and dissipation of heat for the protection of the skin, the cushion must also be viewed as a component of mobility in contributing to trunk stability and as a factor in enhancing performance. The cushion must be as thin as possible to make it easier to reach the wheel handrims, allow the wheelchair to fit under tables, and enhance ease in transfer. Tempered foam that contours to the body shape improves body stability over that provided by lighter foam. Gel-tempered foam combinations, for example, provide more stable support than gel-foam. The gel-tempered foam combines the advantages of trunk stability with heat dissipation. A lower-priced alternative, a composite useful even for heavier weights, is a layer of 2-inch medium foam over a layer of 2-inch hard foam (49,59).

The ability to transfer to and from the wheelchair is an essential component of mobility. Training in independent transfer is possible for persons with good sitting balance. A sliding board is effective provided there is full range of motion at the elbow so it can be mechanically locked in full extension; those with a level of C6 or below can qualify. In addition to a sliding board, fixed overhead loops or a trapeze bar can also be used. This additional equipment requires an overhead frame on the bed, thus limiting its use.

Transfer in and out of an automobile can also be carried out using a sliding board if the car seat is at the same level as the chair. A loop on the wheelchair helps to get the chair in and out of the car without assistance. If this is too taxing, a car-top wheelchair carrier is indicated. A person functioning at a C6 level can thus drive his own car, equipped with hand controls of brakes, power steering, and automatic transmission. A steering device useful for aiding grip strength or wrist flexibility is generally used even by paraplegics, since only one hand is available for steering at any given moment.

The availability of flexion at the elbow permits the person to participate in transfer using a swiveling support attached to a trapeze bar or fixed loops. Assistance is needed in making the swing between the chair and bed. In the absence of elbow flexion (above C5 level), full assistance is required, using a transfer board or a mechanical lift. Vans with power lift, can be driven by someone in a wheelchair, thus extending the range of those able to drive themselves to persons functioning at a C5 level. Servo-assisted steering and braking make it possible for some with shoulder control alone to be independent operators (61,62).

One can consider mobility as extending beyond the ability to get around to encompass participation within a wide range of sports. Technical aids of various kinds and improvements in wheelchairs have permitted a far greater degree of re-entry into the mainstream of life. Examples include snow skiing using either a mono-ski with outriggers or a molded sit-ski as well as modified wheelchairs suitable for marathon racing (63).

Activities of daily living

Activities dealing with personal care that primarily involve hand function are the focus of the occupational therapist. Methods for maximizing upper extremity function in those with quadriplegia include substitution of function, orthoses, and surgical intervention. FES may also in the future contribute to an integrated approach, which frequently will include multiple modalities, such as replacements for the upper extremities, robotics, and trained animals.

As noted earlier, normal sensation—particularly of tactile gnosis—is critical to precise upper extremity function without dependence on visual input alone. A stable shoulder and forearm are the required platform from which hand function must operate. Both muscle strength and full range of motion of the joints are required if the hand is to move into positions where grasp can be useful. Since the goal is increased function, not only the grasp but also the function of the entire arm must be considered as an overall system (Egbert R., personal communication). In recognition of the need for a more functional classification, actual muscle actions are emphasized in the following descriptions, rather than spinal cord neurological levels.

Full range of motion in the neck and at least fair-plus (3+) strength in the neck musculature are required to use a mouth stick effectively. Using a mouth stick, one can accomplish desktop activities such as writing, typing, or reading. It can also be used to operate pushbutton machinery such as telephones, calculators, and environmental control systems. The full range of activities can be expanded enormously by incorporating a robotic arm and computer into the system (64). Voice activation or sip-puff controls can also be used at this level of function to operate devices.

The availability of even very weak proximal upper extremity muscles can be augmented by removing the need to overcome gravity by the use of mobile arm supports—a "ball-bearing feeder" attached to the wheelchair. Hand placement can then be altered despite relatively poor proximal strength, so that, for example, those with poor-minus (2—) strength in the deltoids, biceps, or brachioradialis can accomplish electric wheelchair propulsion, feeding, washing, and grooming, as well as simple desktop and recreational activities. The person must be in an upright position, which requires hip flexion to the range of 95°, and any necessary lateral trunk supports and back support must be in place on the wheelchair. Adequate passive range of motion in the shoulder and forearm increases effectiveness. For example, humeral abduction and flexion of 0–90° will allow full vertical motion of the forearm to head from desk; full elbow flexion to 140° is necessary for hand to mouth activities.

If the hand can be placed where desired by the mobile arm support, feeding utensils, typing sticks, pens, paintbrushes, toothbrushes, hair combs, and many other common devices can be placed in a universal cuff, a 1-inch-wide cuff with a pocket placed around the palm of the hand into which the appropriate utensil is inserted. At this point, the person has become an active contributor to carrying out daily activities, although exact positioning and setup still requires an attendant.

Despite shoulder musculature strong enough to move the upper arm through the range described above and the addition of elbow flexion, the wrist may lack extension, a major component in prehension. The wrist can be stabilized with a static wrist hand orthosis (WHO), which supports the hand in approximately 20° of extension and maintains the thumb's carpal-metacarpal joint in flexion. This maintains the position used in many functional activities and is critical in ensuring optimal recovery should return of the hand musculature occur. Maintaining the abduction range of the thumb is particularly important, since it is necessary should volitional control return or when using a dynamic WHO. Maintenance of the naturally flexed position of the metacarpal-phalangeal (MP) joints allows the development of flexor tendon tightness, a key component of the passive tenodesis grasp wherein finger flexion occurs with wrist dorsiflexion. Although primarily a positional orthosis, the static WHO may, for example, enhance the ability to carry out wheelchair propulsion and can be used in combination with the universal cuff for activities of daily living instead of a dynamic WHO. It cocks the wrist up and provides a place to passively attach utensils and tools of various sorts [see Baumgartner (65) for a fuller description of the training procedures].

To achieve prehension at this level of function, an external source of power must replace the absent wrist extensors. For example, a ratchet WHO maintains the wrist in a static position and stabilizes the thumb with the MP joint abducted in flexion; the thumb is thus aligned with the index and middle fingers. Another portion of the orthosis stabilizes the index and middle fingers in flexion at the interphalangeal joints, permitting pad-to-pad prehension of these fingers with the thumb ("three jaw chuck grasp"). A ratchet mechanism activated by pressure allows the fingers to open or close.

All the so-called tenodesis splints imitate this prototype. The general principle is that a rigid splint captures the forearm, thumb, and index and middle fingers. Jointing of the wrist permits flexion or extension. The thumb is held rigid while the MP joints are hinged. Wrist dorsiflexion flexes the MP joints, and the rigidly held fingers are channeled into a pinch with the opposed thumb. Wrist flexion results in finger extension and release of the grasp.

It is important to recognize that the strength of the grip is limited to 5–10 pounds. The orthosis is difficult to put on and take off, and is easily broken. In addition, it is often considered unsightly. The rate of acceptance and continued usage post-rehabilitation are thus relatively low despite the high initial cost and the need for extensive training. Those persons with fair or better wrist extensors (C6 level) have several options. They may be able to manipulate light objects using only the natural tenodesis grip. Adequate wrist extensor strength permits the use of a wrist-driven WHO to augment the natural tenodesis grip, allowing more power and greater precision in prehension.

Reconstructive hand surgery has its greatest application in those with absent or weak wrist extensors or those with strong wrist extensors whose tenodesis effect does not permit sustained activity. The goal is to enhance the tenodesis effect and not compromise this activity by wrist fusion. A further goal is to achieve key pinch, in which the thumb is in apposition to the radial surface of the index finger. This is a more useful and more easily accomplished goal than the three jaw chuck grasp. Surgery can be considered only after motor and sensory function has reached a plateau (at least 1 year post-injury) (66). Muscles to be considered for transfer must be rated at least 4/5 (MRC scale). Despite adequate strength, spasticity is an absolute contraindication to using a muscle for transfer.

The order of surgery is to begin on the dominant hand if both are classified at the same level. If function is asymmetrical, surgery is done first on the side with the greater function. If there is inadequate cutaneous sensibility, surgery should be done only on the side with the better sensibility. If surgery is to be done to restore elbow extension by deltoid-to-triceps transfer, it should be the first surgical procedure. An active elbow extensor improves the function of a later brachioradialis transfer, since the elbow extensor acts as an antagonist. The action of the brachioradialis in elbow flexion must be overcome for the transplanted muscle to carry out its desired effect of wrist extension. Reconstructive elbow extension is also useful in its own right because it aids in achieving stability in the wheelchair and improves control of the forearm.

Persons with a strong brachioradialis and weak wrist extensor are candidates for transfer so as to provide sufficient strength to dorsiflex the wrist against at least 5 pounds of resistance. One may thus be able to operate a wrist-driven WHO. Moberg (2) describes reconstructive surgery of the hand to achieve a key grip to be done in conjunction with brachioradialis transfer or some other source of strong wrist dorsiflexion. After release of the flexor pollicis longus tendon, it is transferred to the volar surface of the radius. When the wrist goes into active extension, the flexor tenodesis presses the thumb against the side of the index finger, producing a key grip. Fixation of the distal thumb joint with wire prevents the flexion of the interphalangeal joint. There are a number of modifications of this basic operation, depending on an individual's clinical presentation.

In general, the best results have occurred from the least complex operations. Moberg (2) has also emphasized the importance of the hand not only as a tool for manipulation and prehension but also as a basis for human contact. A major goal, therefore, is to keep the hand soft and pliable and to avoid procedures involving the index finger and other digits.

Another option achieving key pinch for tonic activities is via implanted electrodes (67). FES of the finger flexor and thumb adductor can, for example, enable the hand to hold a pen between the index and long fingers, with the thumb serving as a clamp. It is necessary first to bring about increased strength and fatigue resistance by electrically stimulated exercise in those muscles with intact lower motor neuron innervation (68). A more total systematic approach for persons with a neurological level of C5 or C6 might therefore include the combination of orthoses, surgery, and FES as appropriate.

The triceps are available at a neurological level of C7, permitting control of the upper extremity in space with precision in all positions and not limited to sitting. The availability of wrist flexion and finger extensors provides control in manipulating objects. Usually, use of padded handles permits sufficient grip to obviate the need for the use of a prehension splint.

Breathing

The maintenance of adequate ventilation is generally possible so long as the action of the diaphragm remains intact. The ability to carry out a rise in the epigastric area against gravity alone during full inspiration defines a rating of "fair" for that muscle. Retraining and strengthening programs for the diaphragm by resistive exercise can be carried out as with other muscles. Fifty to seventy percent of the pre-injury vital capacity (tidal volume plus inspiratory and expiratory reserve) can be regained despite the loss of the contribution to inspiration by the intercostal muscles in persons with SCI involving cervical lesions (69), in whom expiratory reserve volume is provided by the action of muscles that insert on the upper rib cage. The clavicular portion of the pectoralis major apparently plays a major role, as do the latissimus dorsi and/or teres muscles. The active training of those muscles may therefore increase the capacity to clear secretions (70).

With thoracic lesions, the loss of innervation of the abdominal musculature markedly reduces expiratory reserve. The application of external abdominal pressure to induce coughing and the use of an abdominal binder to increase diaphragmatic efficiency while sitting can substitute for the effects of the absent abdominal wall.

Hypoventilation is defined in those without pre-existing pulmonary disease by P_{CO_2} above 40 and is an indication for mechanical ventilation. Those with a vital capacity of 1,000 ml or less are ventilator dependent. Involvement of the spinal cord at the level of the innervation of the diaphragm (C4 or above) leads to transient or more permanent need for ventilators.

The management of the person requiring a ventilator will not be described in detail here because of its complexity. In general (71), intermittent positive pressure machines provide a preset volume of gas with a tidal volume of 10–15 ml/kg. This higher than "normal" tidal volume has eliminated the need for occasional "sighing" and is more physiologically acceptable to the lung. There is also usually 3–5 cm of H_2O of PEEP (positive end-expiratory pressure) to prevent airway closure. Respiratory rate is maintained in the range of 8–14/min. The positive pressure reduces venous return to the heart and thus cardiac output during inspiration. To reduce this effect, an inspiratory to expiratory ratio of 1:2 is maintained. Weaning procedures may require a return to sensitivity of the respiratory center to CO_2 by a gradual increase in the dead space in the tubing between the ventilator and the lungs, thus increasing the amount of CO_2 rebreathed.

Those whose injury is above the level of innervation of the diaphragm (C2 or above) may have the option of life without the continuous use of a ventilator if the phrenic nerve is intact (72,73). After muscle retraining, chronically implanted electrodes controlled by a transmitter can pace the diaphragm by stimulating one or both phrenic nerves (74).

THE GOALS OF REHABILITATION

Given the character of the neurological impairments and the potential for minimizing the resultant disabilities, it is now necessary to establish the appropriate objectives of an individual's rehabilitation program. The methods used for establishing goals can be an important factor in the ultimate success of any rehabilitation program.

A number of scales are used to measure overall rehabilitation program effectiveness for groups of persons with SCI as well as other physical impairments. Such scales have also been used to assess the effects of any rehabilitation program for specific individuals. The Barthel Index has met with particular acceptance (75). It consists of two parts, a self-care index and a mobility index, with points assessed within each of these categories for individual skills and the level of their performance. If one requires assistance with any one of these skills, the score is variably reduced. For example, "dressing the upper body" within the self-care index is assigned 5 points if the level of performance is "can do by myself" but reduced to 3 points if "can do with help of someone else." Within that same index, "eating" is assigned 6 points if done without any help; and 0 points if any help is required. The total possible score for both categories is 100, with a score greater than 60 signifying relative independence. Using the index in a number of different neurological syndromes, it is particularly interesting that an evaluation of the effect of rehabilitation in 95 persons with SCI showed a median score of 26 at entry and one of 71 at discharge.

Still another measure of effectiveness is the PULSES profile. Although

REHABILITATION

Granger et al. (75) found it overall less sensitive than the Barthels Index for persons with SCI, the acronym reflects portions relevant to SCI dealing with motor function of both the upper and lower limbs and with excretory functions. It also measures the degree of medical supervision required and the degree of environmental support required. Within each category, increased dependence or dysfunction is reflected in an increased score.

More recently, the Quadriplegia Index of Function (QIF) was developed to provide a more sensitive measure of function in the activities of daily living (76). A total score of 100 reflects differential weighting of 10 categories of function. For example, dressing contributes 10 points to the final score whereas feeding can potentially contribute 12 points. Within each category, a fairly large number of specific actions receive an equal number of points. Within the dressing category, for example, the component skills include dressing the upper body, undressing the upper body, socks on, socks off, etc. Within each of these skill areas a total of 4 points is given if done without any assistive device; 3 if done with an assistive device but no human supervision; 2 if it requires human supervision but no lifting; 1 point if lifting is required.

In addition, the QIF contains a questionnaire sampling the level of understanding about such areas as respiratory function, skin breakdown, and urinary tract infection. For example, in the last area, questions deal with signals of infection, what to do if an infection is suspected, and how to prevent infection. The introduction of these questions is particularly innovative. It recognizes the need for development of knowledge during the rehabilitation process necessary to deal with health problems arising out of SCI in the continuing care phase.

Although apparently helpful in assessing the overall effects of a rehabilitation program, none of these scales can adequately reflect the scope of rehabilitation goals that may be appropriate for any one person with SCI (77). "Rehabilitation Indicators" provides the most complete range of possible objectives. Its "Skill Indicators" section contains samples of a large number of areas of function, including self-care and mobility. There appears to be no attempt to rank the various actions within each category but rather to describe a range of activities. For example, there are eight separate descriptors dealing with the use of wheelchairs, including such potential goals as "sitting in wheelchair with head up," "wheeling manually," and "opening doors and passing through" (78).

The most thorough clinically based descriptors that can be used for defining rehabilitation goals are those of Nixon for physical therapy outcomes in SCI (79). Sample goals are provided, with a number of component objectives. For example, an overall goal for the use of the wheelchair is: "Wheelchair-dependent patient demonstrates the ability to direct, assist with, or operate a wheelchair indoors and outdoors." Components include forward/backward turns, safe fall out of wheelchair, and management of all wheelchair parts, etc.

These various scales and sets of descriptors show a continuum of increasing detail in defining the possible goals of any rehabilitation program. However, the actual determination of the goals and ultimately the assessment of the efficacy of any individual's program require still another step. The ordering of priorities in terms of commitment of time and energy, and the relative weights to be assigned to any one goal, cannot be predetermined. Crucial assumptions are being made when feeding is to be assigned more or fewer points than dressing, or when any use of technology or additional help from another person is deemed to be less effective. A choice may be made by one person with SCI to emphasize certain skills over others. Moreover, a decision to use technology and/or a caretaker to deal with certain activities of daily living may make possible a life that includes a job or some other mode of community participation. The determination of an individual's actual disabilities—the significant functional consequences for that person arising out of the impairments—and thus the appropriate objectives for rehabilitation can best be defined with input from the person with the problem.

One may illustrate this individuality in rehabilitation goals in a survey of several men hospitalized with recent injury to their spinal cords in the region of T4-T6. Although their lesions were at the same level with identical consequences in terms of impairment of bowel, bladder, motor and sensory function, their answers to a question about the ways their injury had disabled them were different.

One young man spoke freely without any suggestions needed: "I was six feet four before. Now that I am in a chair, I can't reach the upper shelf or the top of the refrigerator. I look at those things up there and I'm frustrated. I would like to figure out how to get those things down." When asked about any other concerns, he said, "Being in a chair doesn't bother me in other ways. I can wheel along when other people are walking." A middle-aged man had more difficulty in expressing his concern. However, when he was offered several suggestions as to how SCI may have affected others, he chose something related to "not being the man I was." He went on to talk about his feeling of being vulnerable in a wheelchair. "I was the strongest person in my health spa. I didn't try to throw my weight around, but people didn't pick on me the way they did when I was younger. Being in a chair, I think that someone would feel that

REHABILITATION

they could attack me and I would not be able to defend myself." Still another older man expressed freely his concern about being able to work again and support his family.

The appropriate rehabilitation program for each of these persons should reflect their stated needs in concert with the larger categories of mobility, activities of daily living, and so forth. The young man described above would have a high priority for the use of a standing frame and tools for reaching objects at a distance. The middle-aged man might become far more enthusiastic about his training program in transfers if he also enrolled in a weight-lifting body-building program and learned about a karate class for people in wheelchairs. Much more emphasis could be given to designing a vocational program for the third patient.

The determination that disabilities arise only from the characteristics of a person fails to recognize that problems interfering with function may reside elsewhere (80). Architectural barriers and the lack of adaptability of persons in the environment to individuals with SCI may hinder solutions to the problems arising out of the impairments. The nature of the physical and social environments, and such factors as the availability of caretakers, can also affect the goals. Changes can thus be sought not only in the person with impairments but also in the character of the physical environment in terms of ramps and widened doorways and accessible transportation systems.

Technology is particularly useful in increasing the fit between the person and his or her surroundings. Technology in the form of wheelchairs, for example, is more appropriately selected or designed if one adequately defines the problems in terms of both the person—the physical impairments and life goals—and the characteristics of the specific environment (81,82).

The process by which persons with SCI can help define their concerns and goals requires awareness on the part of the professional of a methodology for such participatory planning. The goal is to maximize such participation to increase the likelihood of commitment in carrying out the rehabilitation program. The very process of planning the rehabilitation program—the definition of the problems and the specification of the goals with the maximal participation of the person with SCI—can increase the degree to which the rehabilitation process is effective. One may also enhance the ability of the person to solve not only the problems dealing with rehabilitation but also problems in general. The development of that skill in persons with SCI should be a major goal of any rehabilitation process.

References

1. Moberg E (1978): *The Upper Limb in Tetraplegia: A New Approach to Surgical Rehabilitation.* Stuttgart: Georg Thieme Publishers.
2. Moberg E (1975): Surgical treatment for absent single-hand grip and elbow extension in quadriplegia. *J Bone Joint Surg [Am]* 57:196–206.
3. Donovan W, Dimitrijevic M, Dahm L, Dimitrijevic M (1982): Neurophysiological approaches to chronic pain following spinal cord injury. *Paraplegia* 20:135–146.
4. Welch R, Lobley S, O'Sullivan S, Freed M (1986): Functional independence in quadriplegia: critical levels. *Arch Phys Med Rehab* 67:235–240.
5. Hussey R, Stauffer E (1973): Spinal cord injury: requirements for ambulation. *Arch Phys Med Rehab* 54:544–547.
6. Freehafer A, Vonhaam E, Allen V (1974): Tendon transfers to improve grasp after injuries of the cervical cord. *J Bone Joint Surg* 56A:951.
7. Zancolli E (1975): Surgery for the quadriplegic hand with active strong wrist extension preserved. *Clin Orthop* 112:101.
8. McDowell CL, Moberg EA, Smith AG (1979): International Conference on Surgical Rehabilitation of the Upper Limb in Tetraplegia. *J Hand Surg* 4:390.
9. Hackler R (1984): *Urologic Care of the Spinal Cord Injured Patient,* Lesson 35, vol III. Houston: American Urological Association.
10. Hackler R (1979): Surgical treatment of the adult neurogenic bladder dysfunction. In: *Clinical Neuro-urology,* edited by Krane RJ, Siroky MB. Boston: Little, Brown, pp 197–212.
11. Gunasekera W, Richardson A, Seneviratne K, Eversden I (1984): Clinical correlation of urodynamic findings in patients with localized partial lesions of the spinal cord and cauda equina. *Surg Neurol* 21:148–154.
12. Wein AJ, Raezer DM (1979): Physiology of micturition. In: *Clinical Neuro-urology,* edited by Krane RJ, Siroky MB. Boston: Little, Brown, pp 1–35.
13. Boyarsky S, Labay P, Hanick P, Abramson A, Boyarsky R (1979): *Care of the Patient with Neurogenic Bladder.* Boston: Little, Brown.
14. Krane R, Siroky M (1979): Classification of neuro-urological disorders. In: *Clinical Neuro-urology,* edited by Krane RJ, Siroky MB. Boston: Little, Brown, pp 143–158.
15. Mayo M, Kiviat M (1980): Increased residual urine in patients with bladder neuropathy secondary to suprasacral spinal cord lesions. *J Urol* 123:726–728.
16. Khanna OP (1979): Non-surgical therapeutic modalities. In: *Clinical Neuro-urology,* edited by Krane RJ, Siroky MB. Boston: Little, Brown, pp 159–196.
17. Pavlakis A, Siroky M, Goldstein I, Krane R (1983): Neurological findings in conus medullaris and cauda equina injury. *Arch Neurol* 40:570–573.
18. Guttmann L (1959): The regulation of rectal function in spinal paraplegia. *Proc Royal Soc Med* 52:86.

19. Frankel H (1967): Bowel training. *Paraplegia* 4:254–256.
20. Haymaker W (1956): *Bing's Local Diagnosis in Neurological Diseases*. St. Louis: C. V. Mosby.
21. Nathan P, Smith M (1953): Spinal pathways subserving defecation and sensation from the lower bowel. *J Neurol Neurosurg Psychiatry* 16:245–256.
22. Connell A, Frankel H, Guttmann L (1963): The motility of the pelvic colon following complete lesions of the spinal cord. *Paraplegia* 1:98–115.
23. Melzack J, Porter N (1963): Studies on the reflex activity of the external sphincter ani in man. *Paraplegia* 1:277–296.
24. Denny-Brown D, Robertson E (1935): An investigation of the nervous control of defecation. *Brain* 58:256–310.
25. Trieschmann RB (1980): *Spinal Cord Injuries: Psychological, Social and Vocational Adjustment*. New York: Pergamon Press, pp 127–146.
26. Siroky MB, Krane RJ (1979): Physiology of male sexual function. In: *Clinical Neuro-urology*, edited by Krane RJ, Siroky MB. Boston: Little, Brown, pp 45–62.
27. Rivard DJ (1982): Anatomy, physiology, and neurophysiology of male sexual function. In: *Management of Male Impotence*, edited by Bennett AH. Baltimore: William & Wilkins, pp 1–25.
28. Comarr A (1971): Sexual concepts in traumatic cord and cauda equina lesions. *J Urol* 106:375–378.
29. Comarr A, Vigue M (1978): Sexual counselling among male and female patients with spinal cord and/or cauda equina injury. Part I. *Am J Phys Med* 57:107–122.
30. Comarr A, Vigue M (1978): Sexual counselling among male and female patients with spinal cord and/or cauda equina injury. Part II. *Am J Phys Med* 57:215–227.
31. Comarr A (1985): Sexuality and fertility among spinal cord and/or cauda equina injuries. *J Am Paraplegia Soc* 8:67–74.
32. Guttmann L, Walsh J (1971): Prostigmin assessment test of fertility in spinal man. *Paraplegia* 9:39.
33. Nance P, Gwner M, Nance D (1983): Gonadal regulation in men with flaccid paraplegia. *Arch Phys Med Rehab* 64:757–759.
34. Yalla SV (1982): Sexual dysfunction in the paraplegic and quadriplegic. In: *The Management of Male Impotence*, edited by Bennett AH. Baltimore: Williams & Wilkins.
35. Stjernberg L, Blumberg H, Wallin B (1986): Sympathetic activity in man after spinal cord injury: outflow to muscle below the lesion. *Brain* 109:695–715.
36. Guttmann L (1973): *Spinal Cord Injuries: Comprehensive Management and Research*. London: Blackwell Scientific Publishers.
37. Wolf E, Magora A (1976): Orthostatic and ergometric evaluation of cord injured patients. *Scand J Rehab Med* 8:93–96.

38. Fryschuss V, Knuttson E (1969): Cardiovascular control in man with transverse cervical cord lesions. *Life Sci* 8:421–424.
39. Wallin B, Stjernberg L (1984): Sympathetic activity in man after spinal cord injury: outflow to skin below the lesion. *Brain* 107:183–198.
40. Rossier A, Fam B, Lee I (1982): Role of striated and smooth muscle components in the urethral pressure profile in traumatic neurogenic bladders. *J Urol* 128:529–535.
41. Yalla SV (1979): Spinal cord injury. In: *Clinical Neuro-urology,* edited by Krane RJ, Siroky MB. Boston: Little, Brown, pp 229–244.
42. Phillips L, Ozer MN, Axelson P (1987): *A Guide to Spinal Cord Injury for Patients and Their Families.* New York: Raven Press.
43. Kolodny RC, Masters WH, Johnson VE (1979): *Textbook of Sexual Medicine.* Boston: Little, Brown.
44. Nadig PW, Ware JC, Blumoff R (1986): Non-invasive device to produce and maintain an erection-like state. *Urology* 27:126–131.
45. Furlow WL (1979): Therapy of impotence. In: *Clinical Neuro-urology,* edited by Krane RJ, Siroky MB. Boston: Little, Brown.
46. Sidi AA, Lange PH (1986): Recent advances in the diagnosis and management of impotence. *Urol Clin North Am* 13:489–500.
47. Constantian MB, Jackson HS (1980): Biology and care of the pressure sore wound. In: *Pressure Ulcers: Principles and Technique of Management,* edited by Constantian MB. Boston: Little, Brown, p 69.
48. Eriksson E (1980): Etiology: microcirculatory effects of pressure. In: *Pressure Ulcers: Principles and Technique of Management,* edited by Constantian MB. Boston: Little, Brown, p 7.
49. Ferguson-Pell M, Cochran G, Palmieri V, Buinski J (1986): Development of a modular wheelchair cushion for spinal cord injured persons. *J Rehab Res Dev* 23:63–76.
50. Redford JB (1987): Orthotics. In: *Physical Medicine and Rehabilitation State of the Art Reviews,* vol 1, no 1. Philadelphia: Hanley and Belfus.
51. Cybulski G, Penn R, Jaeger R (1984): Lower extremity electrical stimulation in cases of spinal cord injury. *Neurosurgery* 15:132–146.
52. Kralj A, Jaeger R (1982): Posture switching enables prolonged standing in paraplegic patients functionally electrically stimulated. In: *Proceedings of 5th Annual Conference on Rehabilitation Engineering.* Washington, D.C.: RESNA.
53. Waters R, McNeal D, Perry J (1975): Experimental correction of footdrop by electrical stimulation of peroneal nerve. *J Bone Joint Surg [Am]* 57:1047–1054.
54. Jaeger R, Kralj A (1983): Studies in functional electrical stimulation for standing and forward progression. In: *Proceedings of 6th Annual Conference on Rehabilitation Engineering.* Washington, D.C.: RESNA.
55. Marsolais E, Kobetic R, Cockoff G, Peckham P (1983): Reciprocal walking in paraplegic patients using internal functional electrical stimulation. *Pro-*

ceedings of 6th Annual Conference on Rehabilitation Engineering. Washington, D.C.: RESNA.
56. Miller N, Merkel K, Merritt J (1985): Leg braces: efficiency and energy expenditure. *J Am Paraplegia Soc* 8:75–79.
57. Peterson MJ (1985): Ambulation and orthotic management. In: *Spinal Cord Injury,* edited by Adkins HV. New York: Churchill Livingstone, pp 199–218.
58. Clinkingbeard J, Gersten J, Hoehn D (1964): Energy cost of ambulation in the traumatic paraplegic. *Am J Phys Med* 43:157–165.
59. Edberg E, Adkins HV (1985): Wheelchairs and cushions. In: *Spinal Cord Injury,* edited by Adkins HV. New York: Churchill Livingstone, pp 177–197.
60. Brubaker C (1986): Wheelchair prescription: an analysis of factors that affect mobility and performance. *J Rehab Res Dev* 23:19–26.
61. Alvarez SE (1985): Functional assessment and training. In: *Spinal Cord Injury,* edited by Adkins HV. New York: Churchill Livingstone, pp 131–155.
62. Less M, Colverd EG, DeMauro GE, Young J (1978): *Teaching Driver Education to the Physically Disabled.* Albertson, NY: Human Resources Center.
63. Kegel B (1985): Physical fitness: sports and recreation for those with lower limb amputation or impairment. *J Rehab Res Dev* Clinical Supplement 1.
64. Seamone W, Schmeisser G (1985): Early clinical evaluation of a robot/arm worktable system for spinal cord injured persons. *J Rehab Res Dev* 22:38–57.
65. Baumgarten JM (1978): Upper extremity adaptations for the person with quadriplegia. In: *Spinal Cord Injury,* edited by Adkins HV. New York: Churchill Livingstone, p 225.
66. McDowell CL (1981): Tetraplegia. In: *Operative Hand Surgery,* edited by Green DP. New York: Churchill Livingstone, pp 1109–1127.
67. Peckham P, Mortimer J, Marsolais E (1980): Controlled prehension and release in the C5 quadriplegic elicited by functional electrical stimulation of the paralyzed forearm musculature. *Ann Biomed Eng* 8:369–388.
68. Peckham P, Mortimer J, Marsolais E (1976): Upper and lower motor neuron lesions in the upper extremity muscles of tetraplegics. *Paraplegia* 14:115–121.
69. Wetzel J (1985): Respiratory evaluation and treatment. In: *Spinal Cord Injury,* edited by Adkins HV. New York: Churchill Livingstone, pp 75–98.
70. DeTroyer A, Estenne M, Heilporn A (1986): *New Engl J Med* 314:740–744.
71. Stonnington H (1980): Respirators and respiratory aids. In: *Orthotics etcetera,* edited by Redford JB. Baltimore: Williams & Wilkins, p 563.
72. Markand O, Kincaid J, Pourmand R, Moorthy S (1984): Electrophysiologic evaluation of diaphragm by transcutaneous phrenic nerve stimulation. *Neurology* 34:604–614.
73. Shaw R, Glenn W, Hogan J, Phelps M (1980): Electrophysiological evalua-

tion of phrenic nerve function in candidates for diaphragm pacing. *J Neurosurg* 53:345–354.
74. Glenn W, Holcomb W, Shaw R, Hogan J, Holschuk K (1976): Long term ventilatory support by diaphragm pacing in quadriplegia. *Ann Surg* 183:566.
75. Granger C, Albrecht G, Hamilton B (1979): Outcome of comprehensive medical rehabilitation: measurement by PULSES profile and the Barthel Index. *Arch Phys Med Rehab* 60:145–151.
76. Gresham G, Labi M, Dittmar S, Hicks J, Joyce S, Strelik M (1986): The quadriplegia index of function (QIF). *Paraplegia* 24:38–44.
77. *Functional Limitations: A State of the Art Review.* Falls Church, VA: Indices, Inc.
78. Diller L, Fordyce W, Jacobs D, Brown M (1979): *Rehabilitation Indicators: Overview and Forms.* New York: New York University Press.
79. Nixon V (1985): *Spinal Cord Injury: A Guide to Functional Outcome in Physical Therapy Management.* Rockville, MD: Aspen.
80. DeJong G (1980): What's different about functional assessment in independent living? In: *Symposium on Functional Limitations*, edited by Turner R. Cambridge, MA: Abt Associates, Inc.
81. Ozer M (1986): The design process viewed as a technology. In: *Proceedings of the 9th Annual Conference on Rehabilitation Technology.* Washington, D.C.: RESNA/AART.
82. Ozer M (1988): A methodology for wheelchair selection: a participatory planning process. *J Rehab Res Dev* Special Supplement 2 (in press).

CHAPTER **4**

Continuing Care

The major goal of the acute care phase was to safeguard the spinal cord to minimize impairment resulting from injury, whereas in the rehabilitation phase the goal was to minimize disability in light of continued impairment. During the continuing care phase, the focus shifts again. The aim is now to maximize health—the ability to function effectively both in body and in spirit within the community. The methods for collecting information for the accomplishment of this goal also change.

During the acute and rehabilitation phases, the neurological examination is the major technique for defining the character of the impairment. At the outset, it localizes the areas of injury and provides the basis for clinical decisions as to surgical intervention. Subsequently, it provides a basis for determining the functional consequences of injury— the disabilities. The aspects of the neurological examination used for the latter differs somewhat from that used for localization. For example, there may be greater concern for the sensory aspects of the examination, for specific salient muscle actions directly related to activities such as self-care, transfer, and ambulation, and for autonomic functions.

The definition of the disabilities heavily, but not entirely, depends on the character of the impairments. As discussed previously, the definition of the disabilities and thus the goals for rehabilitation require input from the person with the problem as well as the objective signs derived from the neurological examination. During the continuing care phase, this trend becomes even more evident. The management of the continuing or late effects of the initial injury requires ongoing and an even greater degree of participation by the person with the problem.

The change that occurs in this phase is the *degree* to which the person with SCI functions on his own. The person with SCI is not necessarily "ill" by virtue of SCI, but an increased likelihood of significant medical problems requires vigilance. Information must be generated by the patient independently of the health care professionals as to when a problem exists that requires attention, how to act to deal with this problem alone to the extent possible, and when to seek medical help.

One goal of rehabilitation then should be to help the person understand that specific indicators may be used to identify the existence of illness, and that these signals may well be different from those used in the past. It becomes important to help the person recognize that the injury has changed some of the ways in which his body reacts.

The person with SCI becomes a major resource in managing his own health care, learning to identify what are his or her own specific characteristics and thus increasingly contributing to the understanding by the professional of appropriate diagnosis and treatment. This becomes particularly important in light of changes with age and other factors as one's body interacts with the initial set of impairments. It is clear that this identification process becomes important in the management of the urinary tract, the skin, and other systems particularly susceptible to illness (1). Total care of the person with SCI requires that such learning be an integral part of the health care process. The application of this same approach to some prototype neurological problems further illustrates this principle.

Problems in Continuing Care

Post-traumatic syringomyelia

The syndrome is one of dissociated sensory loss and the development of a lower motor neuron deficit following a previously stable lesion. The incidence of such progressive neurological impairment secondary to post-traumatic cyst formation within the spinal cord varies. One recent study establishes a higher incidence than previously reported, of 7.2% in those with complete tetraplegia (2). There is considerable unpredictability in the time elapsed between the initial injury and the identification of this complication. The average time from injury to appearance of symptoms was in the range of 10 years for those with incomplete lesions and 4 years for those with complete lesions.

The intramedullary enlargement, lined by glial tissue, extends from the area of myelomalacia in the initial area of injury, with enlargement sometimes occurring precipitously in response to changes in intracranial pressure. However, postmortem examination generally shows no direct connection between the cyst and the subarachnoid space. Cyst enlargement is presumably due to some other mechanism such as seepage along the perivascular spaces (3).

These changes can lead to dramatic functional consequences in persons who already have major disabilities (4). The availability of surgical treatment to arrest further progression via long-term drainage of the cyst has lent some urgency to its early identification. A "bullseye" on delayed CT following metrizamide myelography has been a relatively sensitive and specific diagnostic finding (5). Even more recently, early identification by noninvasive magnetic resonance imaging (MRI) has increased the understanding of the natural history of this condition and the significance of its differentiation from myelomalacia per se (6).

The mode of presentation of the cyst varies with the underlying spinal cord involvement. Growth of the cyst below the level of the lesion may reduce hyperreflexia and convert an upper motor neuron bladder to that of a lower motor neuron. The ascent of findings above the level of the initial lesion is more common. In those with confirmed syrinx, the most frequent initial complaint was pain. Its quality, distribution, frequency, and duration vary considerably. It is usually above the site of the original injury but may be below it. Pain is usually aggravated by straining and in some cases is much worse when sitting. There is a variable interval after the appearance of this pain before loss of sensation occurs above the level of the lesion, the next most common mode of presentation (2). Another mode of presentation is that of excess sweating in the area of sensory loss below the level of the injury (7).

The classic finding on neurological examination of relative sparing of light touch reflects the diffuse distribution of fibers subserving touch, with the involvement of both crossed and uncrossed fibers and considerable overlap. The may be relative loss of pain and temperature sensations and/or deep pain, with the latter leading to Charcot-type joints. Even more frequent is a dissociation between loss of pain and the relative sparing of proprioception. The involvement of the caudal portion of the spinal tract of the trigeminal nerve subserving pain and temperature in the face, with touch subserved by the main sensory nucleus in the brainstem, is felt to account for the occasional sensory dissociation in the face.

Motor changes are generally late to appear. An increase in spasticity was an early symptom in some. More frequently, coincident with the sensory changes, loss of deep tendon reflexes may be an early sign indicating involvement of the anterior horn cells (8). In the cervical region, it is difficult to distinguish a new loss of motor function from underlying pathology. Electrodiagnostic studies may show a decrease in the interference pattern and an increase in motor unit amplitude and duration as early signs. Prolongation of the F-wave latencies and their shortening subsequent to drainage of the cyst and improvement in motor function are related to the presence of interstitial edema in the area of the anterior horn cells (9).

Nerve conduction studies typically show maintenance of a normal sensory action potential in the face of loss of sensation on examination and the decrease in the amplitude of the motor response. The sensory action potential remains unaffected, since sensory impairment from a syrinx is a function of the connection between the sensory tracts and the sensory fibers proximal to the dorsal root ganglion, and the dorsal root cell and body are intact. Reduction in the sensory nerve action potential thus suggests peripheral nerve entrapment as a not uncommon additional finding in persons with long-standing SCI (9).

The presenting symptoms and findings on neurological examination aid in determining whether or not a syrinx exists and its presumed site or level, and in deciding to seek confirmation via CT or MRI. The availability of MRI as a noninvasive method of documenting the existence of cysts may well change our understanding of the natural history of this condition. Even with the diagnostic methods used in the past, there has been evidence for the lack of progression of documented cysts (2). The indications for surgery even in the presence of a cyst must relate to the functional consequences of the impairments—to the disabilities resulting from the loss of motor function and to severe pain. The following cases illustrate the need for defining the problem in functional terms rather than merely in terms of the existence of the cyst per se.

CASE REPORTS

H. S. is a 61-year-old man injured 40 years ago in a diving accident. His neurological motor level was C7. His lesion was incomplete, with intact sensation to light touch to the toes. He noted an increase in spasms of both lower extremities, more on the left than the right. The spasms interfered with his ability to sit in his wheelchair without taking precautions against falling. He had no response to an increase in medication. There was no change in sensation above or below the level of the lesion. Delayed CT following metrizamide myelography was suggestive of syrinx at C5, later confirmed on MRI. The degree of disability that could be attributed to the syrinx was not felt by the patient to be significant enough to consent to surgery. More thorough evaluation led to the discovery of a femoral neck fracture whose subsequent healing reduced his spasms to the extent that medication was effective in enabling him to regain his previous ease in sitting.

D. L. is a 35-year-old man injured 11 years ago. His neurological motor level was C7 on the right and C6 on the left. His lesion was incomplete, with touch intact several levels below the motor level. He complained of recent worsening of spasticity in the lower extremities that was unresponsive to medication and interfered with the ability to sit in his chair. He sought the installation of an epidural stimulator as a new mode of treatment. As part of the workup prior to installation, an MRI identified a cyst at C5. In light of this finding, the epidural stimulator was not felt to be indicated. The initial complaint of increased spasticity has become less prominent with a more concerted medical regimen. However, he continues to complain of pain in the shoulder and neck, greater on the left than on the right. The pain is not seriously disabling to him at this time and has responded somewhat to nonsteroidal anti-inflammatory medication. Despite the documented cyst, the decision for surgical drainage has been postponed with the patient's fully informed consent and commitment to monitoring his neurological status in collaboration with the SCI unit.

In the first case, the finding of a cyst might be considered to be a false positive in light of the lack of symptoms that could actually be attributed to its presence. The value of conservative management has been confirmed. The second case illustrates the protean quality of presentation and the need to consider the possibility of a cyst when there has been a change in degree of disability. The availability of MRI increases even more the significance of informed patient participation in decisions for intervention and in ongoing monitoring of symptoms.

The management of spasticity

The management of spasticity in the person with SCI can be clarified by once again distinguishing between the impairments defined by the neurological examination and the disabilities as defined in discussions with the person with SCI. Signs of an upper motor neuron lesion such as hyperreflexia, clonus, and velocity-dependent resistance to passive muscle stretch are indicators of the development of reflex actions independent of supraspinal controls. They are important harbingers for the return of reflex bladder, bowel, and sexual functions. These findings on neurological examination are also useful for localizing the lesion as within the central nervous system; and the level above which the lesion has occurred. They are felt to be indicators of disinhibition of the stretch reflex (10).

However, the major disabilities resulting from the loss of supraspinal controls result from disinhibition of flexor reflexes in the lower limbs rather than disinhibition of the stretch reflex. Flexor reflex afferents are no longer subject to tonic inhibition from the brainstem by the dorsal reticulospinal pathway, with the Babinski-type response associated with isolation of this tract from supraspinal controls (10).

The resulting disabilities described by persons with SCI are problems such as trouble maintaining sitting balance in the wheelchair, interference with transfer from the chair, or difficulty in maintaining control of a powered chair. The signs of spasticity found on neurological examination do not necessarily define the existence of these functional difficulties.

When the spinal cord is deprived of supraspinal control, a large increase in motorneuron activity is manifested as "spasms," or prolonged uncontrolled excessive contractions of skeletal muscles and as pathological responses to stimulation. These spasms can overcome the usual reciprocal relationship between agonists and antagonists within a limb as well as between limbs (11). Particularly relevant to the disabilities experienced are the changes in the response to noxious cutaneous stimuli (12,13). The flexion response to cutaneous stimuli in the lower extremity—the flexor or withdrawal reflex—has its threshold reduced and its receptive field enlarged.

When one touches a hot surface or electrical stimulation is applied to the lower extremity, the person with an intact spinal cord exhibits a flexor reflex. Following SCI, brisk flexor reflexes can be produced by more natural non-noxious stimuli that do not commonly produce flexor movements in normal subjects. If these movements are produced by even less obvious stimuli, they are called flexor spasms. These spasms are indistinguishable from flexor reflexes aside from their lowered threshold. They presumably arise from spinal afferent input, since dorsal rhizotomy can eliminate them. Their frequency is much higher during periods when the limb is the site of a pressure ulcer or other presumed source of noxious afferent stimuli, irrespective of the person's awareness of pain (14).

Flexor spasms are extremely variable and range from brief, repetitive firing of a single motor unit without any visible contraction to sustained firing of many motor units with massive movements. It is not clear why some persons with SCI develop flexor spasms and others do not. Those with flexor spasms appear to have even lower thresholds for the response to non-noxious stimuli than do those without spasms, but there is no quantitative data in this regard (15).

If these spasms are due to a markedly increased response to afferent input, proper management would be to decrease as much of the afferent activity to the cord as possible by avoiding pressure sores, distension, and/or infection of the bladder. More fixed contractures that could preclude sitting and standing ("paraplegia in flexion") can be prevented by facilitating extensor activity through proper positioning and change in position during the acute care and rehabilitative phases. Extensor activity is facilitated by placement in the prone position and, when supine, placement of the limbs in abduction and extension at the hips and the knees (16).

During the continuing care phase, an increase in spasms can be a nonspecific sign of such underlying problems as abscess formation or a bladder problem. Proper management involves a search for such causes and their removal. More frequently, the management of spasms during this phase deals with the symptomatic treatment of the disabilities arising from the spasms themselves. It is important to recognize the appropriate goals of treatment, which is not necessarily or even frequently the removal of the spasticity per se. For example, some persons with SCI find it helpful to use their spasms, and have evolved specific triggers to use them to help turn themselves in bed, or in the process of transfer. For others, the spasticity has been useful for maintaining muscle tone and muscle bulk in their paralyzed extremities. The problem must be defined in terms of the disabilities that spasms create in the context of the person's own life.

The character of the problem caused by the spasms, i.e., the actual disabilities, will vary depending on the interaction between the individual's neurological status and his social and physical environment. The problem can best be defined in collaboration with the person experiencing the spasms. For example, one young man with intact sensation to deep pressure below the level of his cervical lesion had several concerns, including "tightness" in the muscles of his legs associated with the motor spasms and occasionally being thrown out of his chair. He perceived the feeling of tightness as being most troublesome. Another person was concerned when his spasms involved not only his legs but also his abdominal muscles and back. He was afraid that he might hurt his feet on the footrests of his wheelchair when they came to rest after a major spasm. He was particularly concerned that he might fall out of his chair when these unpredictable spasms came on days when his wife worked a day shift and he sat up at home alone.

There may be variation in the times when the spasms are disabling. One man with quadriplegia described his problem to be in the morning, when he found it difficult to remain in his chair while being bathed by his attendant. During the rest of the day he was meeting his criterion of "being able to drive his power chair without losing control." Indeed, he welcomed spasms that occurred during the night, since he used them to help himself turn to relieve pressure. Another man found his spasms more troublesome at night when his moving about in bed interfered with his mate's sleep. Still another was even more specific in defining his problem. He found that spasms were more likely on the several evenings each week just prior to emptying his bowels. He was particularly concerned on those nights about hitting the hot radiator in his bathroom while transferring from the wheelchair to his commode.

Once the problem has been defined in these more functional terms, the goals for treatment can be more appropriately established. For the man with quadriplegia described above, his stated goal, not now being met, was "to remain in my chair without being thrown out while carrying out my early morning self-care." He also wished to maintain his existing level of acceptable function during the remainder of the day and evening. Since he was already on large doses of several medications, his additional goal was to achieve this improvement without increasing the total dosage of medication, and perhaps to decrease it.

A clear statement of the goals leads to their being more frequently achieved or, at the least, being more likely to be noted when achievement did occur. Further, the very process of describing these various goals, in his own words to the extent possible, provides the basis for a person to become a more active as well as more accurate participant in evaluating the efficacy of a treatment. In each case, the measure of effectiveness of treatment can be defined in clinical terms that are meaningful to both the patient and the physician.

TREATMENT

The treatment modalities that aid in managing disabilities due to spasms are similarly most likely to be effective when developed in collaboration with the person with the problem. The effectiveness of any medication can be enhanced when it is part of a more total approach to treatment including, for example, the use of a passive range of motion of the affected muscles, exercise, and heat as described in the subsequent case reports. Even when one deals with medication per se, different individuals may require quite different drug combinations for optimal therapeutic effects. The selection of the proper drug or combination, the selection of the proper dosage, and the proper time for administration can all enhance the effectiveness of the therapy. The knowledge for such decisions can optimally come both from the physician's awareness of neurophysiology and pharmacology and input from the person with the problem, who becomes a major contributor to the evaluation of efficacy.

The effects of the most common classes of drugs appear to be complementary. On the basis of both neurophysiological (17) and pharmacological studies (18), three separate types of drugs can be identified. Their effects seem to be related to no distinct pathophysiological mechanism and may differ in each individual case.

The benzodiazepines, of which diazepam is the prime example, are capable of re-establishing the normal inhibition by tonic vibratory stimuli of monosynaptic reflexes such as the H-reflex (17). This supports its probable primary role within the spinal cord, restoring at least in part the presynaptic inhibition for which the proposed inhibitor is GABA (18). Diazepam is well absorbed orally. Due to its high lipid solubility, it has a rather fast onset of action and wide distribution within the central nervous system. It has a long half-life (50 hours) due to metabolites developed in the liver and its wide distribution throughout the body.

Unlike diazepam, baclofen does not re-establish the effects of tonic vibratory inhibition. It does produce significant changes in electrically evoked flexor reflexes (14). In addition to longer intervals between spontaneous flexor spasms, it causes a rise in the apparent threshold for production of flexor reflexes due to mechanical or electrical stimulation, changing both the latency of the response and its amplitude. It is postulated to reduce the facility with which ordinary afferent input produces flexor responses. Its action therefore appears to be on polysynaptic interneurons. It is rapidly absorbed from the GI tract, with a peak concentration at 2 hours and a mean half-life of 3.5 hours (range, 2.5–6.0). Seventy to eighty percent is excreted in the urine. Only small amounts cross the blood–brain barrier, but mental changes can be detected, particularly in the elderly (19).

Dantrolene is unique among these drugs in that it apparently works at the periphery. It inhibits the release of calcium at the level of the muscle fiber, preventing activation of the contractile apparatus and diminishing the force of contraction. The effect is more pronounced in fast contracting rather than the slower contracting muscles used for postural maintenance (18). It is absorbed rather slowly, with a peak concentration at 5 hours and a half-life in the range of 8–9 hours. It is also substantially bound to albumin. Its metabolites are excreted in the urine. Adverse reactions include muscle weakness, which is associated with the therapeutic actions of the drug, and evidence of liver damage.

The effects of a collaborative management program can be illustrated by the persons whose problems were described earlier. The man whose problem was spasms just before carrying out his bowel program was able to achieve control by taking a single 5-mg dose of diazepam approximately 2 hours before attempting transfer. He did not require medication at any other time. The person with nocturnal spasms found it helpful to take a warm bath prior to sleep. He also found that he did well on those nights when he had bowled, and achieved relief with 10 mg of baclofen on those nights when he had not. He chose not to use diazepam because of his concern about its other central nervous system effects.

The man with quadriplegia described earlier found it helpful to have passive range of motion immediately after arising. Since he was meeting his goals during the afternoon and night, the dosage of both baclofen and diazepam at noon and bedtime were progressively reduced while the amount taken in the early morning was increased. He gradually met his goal of "not falling out of the chair" and retained his already acceptable level of performance throughout the 24-hour period. The dosage was one-third of the original total. He also noted deterioration in performance on mornings when there had been a rapid change in temperature. On those mornings, he would increase his diazepam very slightly, since he found its onset and effects more consistent than those of baclofen. Throughout this period, it was he who defined the degree to which he was achieving his goal. He had become an active participant in his own treatment in collaboration with the physician.

This approach led not only to an increase in the effectiveness of a given amount of medication, but to the very process of having the person with SCI help specify the drug regimen, providing an experience that extended to other aspects of his medical management, including treatment of the skin and genitourinary system. He had become a more informed observer and could begin to define his problems and set goals in these other important areas of function as well.

Intelligent management of medication is further illustrated by the case of a physician with paraplegia whose nocturnal flexor spasms interfered with his sleep (20). Since he found diazepam caused morning lassitude, he chose baclofen to improve his sleep. He finally achieved his goal without side-effects albeit with a total 24-hour dose of 180 mg on a schedule of 20 mg every 2–4 hours. The night-time control persisted even when the dosage was tapered to 80 mg while maintaining a schedule of every 3–4 hours. He found it important to maintain a relatively high frequency of the drug while reducing the amount at each

CONTINUING CARE   97

time. When, for no apparent reason, the night-time spasms returned, he merely temporarily adjusted the total to 100 mg with immediate excellent results.

The author's conclusion was that the effectiveness of the medication was enhanced by his being educated regarding his management. In the case of this physician, education had been self-education, but in the other cases described, it arose in the context of the physician–patient interaction. Chapter 5 deals with the procedures of the planning process used in the cases described earlier. It can be applied as a more generic approach to the management of a variety of problems in both the rehabilitation and continuing care phases.

The management of chronic pain

Pain in persons with SCI is closely allied with the flexor spasms described in the previous section. One may precede, substitute, or follow the other. For example, it is not uncommon during the continuing care phase that worsening of the existing level of spasms signals the appearance of a source of stimuli that would ordinarily lead to a sense of injury or pain in those with an intact spinal cord. Pressure ulcers, an infected toenail, or other sources of injury need to be sought. Spasms thus can substitute for what would be construed as pain if there were not disconnection from conscious awareness.

Pain can also precede the development of spasms, so that distinguishing the order of appearance can be helpful in terms of appropriate treatment. One example is a man whose primary complaint was pain in his back at the level of his spinal fusion. Only after further questioning did it become apparent that the pain would be present for about a minute before spasms of his legs occurred. These spasms would be the proximate cause of his being thrown out of his chair or being awakened at night. Appropriate treatment of the spasms was to deal with the antecedent pain rather than to use medication directed at the spasms per se.

Conversely, the treatment of spasms can alleviate pain. Recall the man described in the previous section with an incomplete cervical lesion and intact sensation to deep pressure in his legs. When asked about his major concern with his spasms, he identified the painful tightening of his leg muscles as particularly troublesome. For him, the treatment of the spasms with medications such as diazepam or baclofen was helpful in alleviating the pain.

Pain can also be attributed to problems above the lesion such as contractures and shoulder involvement, to the level of the lesion in the area of root involvement or associated with movement, or below the level of the lesion (21). The focus in this section is on the sources of pain that may be attributed to the level of the lesion or below, such as diffusely localized burning, tingling sensations. These sensations are referred either to the lower limbs or to some other more specific otherwise "insensitive" areas such as the feet, toes, or anogenital region.

The relationship of these sensations to impairment in response to pinprick in those same areas is unclear. Anterior commissural myelotomy used to treat pain associated with cancer cuts the decussating spinothalamic and the spinoreticulothalamic fibers. The findings in those persons illustrate the complexity of the relationships between clinical pain and sensibility in testing during the neurological examination (22). As an example, in one case autopsy confirmed histological evidence of complete division of the decussating spinothalamic fibers subserving pain and temperature. Post-myelotomy, initial pain relief had been followed by a gradual return of symptoms in the six months before death. Despite the relief from pain, there was at no time any diminution of response to pinprick. Another person had an initial loss of both response to pinprick and deep pain. The response to deep pain remained absent, and pinprick sensibility returned sometime after the return of clinical pain. Still another person had severe pain in the right groin and thigh extending to the knee. Myelotomy was followed by both sensory loss and pain relief during the 6 months prior to death. The relief of pain and the findings of response to pinprick on sensory examination thus appear to be dissociated.

The relationship between impaired sensibility and the existence of symptoms attributed to pain may be further obscured by the limited character of the clinical neurological examination. One measure of the completeness of the cord transection is the discrimination of sharpness from dullness. Despite the lack of response to pinprick under standard conditions, some persons report sensations that are unpleasant or painful when various stimuli are provided either repetitively or in multiple sites simultaneously. These sensations are poorly localized and may appear after a delay or remain after the source of stimulation disappears (23). They replicate the symptoms found below the level of the lesion in many persons who have been considered to have a complete transection of the spinal cord on the basis of the ordinary clinical examination.

The qualities of sensation tested in the classic clinical examination fall for the most part within the faster, larger fibers. Sensations requiring more intense or prolonged stimulation may reflect the characteristics of transmission in the slow or small fibers. It is thus necessary to carry out a more complete neurological examination that samples the function of the slower fibers with repetitive or slow stroking. Another method for amplifying the standard examination is the use of somatosensory evoked response to sample fast fiber transmission.

On the basis of the description of the pain and the findings on the amplified neurological examination, four major categories of chronic pain of unexplained origin in persons with SCI are 1) segmental or radicular, 2) spinal cord or central, 3) visceral, and 4) muscular. The first is generally present since the time of injury, occurs in waves, and is stabbing in character with an undertone of burning or aching. Its distribution is roughly segmental, aggravated by rest and alleviated by activity. Although sensibility to pinprick may not be evident on standard examination, there may be retained slow fiber activity. The spinal cord central pain syndrome may take several months to appear, is relatively constant, and has a tingling or numbing quality. Its distribution is mainly in the distal extremities, aggravated by activity and relieved by rest or solitude. There may be continued evidence of fast fiber activity and thus an incomplete syndrome on standard examination. The visceral type usually appears within a few weeks or months, is generally constant but somewhat variable, and burning in quality. It is poorly localized within the abdominal or pelvic area. The physiological basis remains obscure but is presumably related to slow fiber afferents carried within the autonomic system. Still another very frequent type of pain is associated with muscle tension and movement. It is present mainly at the level of the lesion, particularly in relation to surgery. Pain is aching in quality and is relieved by rest.

Although the degree and type of impairment may vary, even more variable is the degree to which pain may be disabling even in light of the similarity of impairment. The definition of disabling pain differs. One survey (24) defined pain as "moderate" if it is annoying enough for the person to use medication or to modify his behavior somewhat to relieve discomfort, such as going to bed. "Severe" pain is difficult to bear; the person is unable to divert attention from it and is unable to pursue daily activities when the pain is present.

In a randomly selected group of persons with SCI of at least 1 year's duration, the most frequent complaint was of "burning" pain below the level of the lesion. Approximately half of these had their symptoms categorized as either moderate or severe, with the latter 15% of the total. Aching type pain at the level of the lesion was next in frequency; 75% of these had some disability and 25% had severe pain. Radicular shooting pain was less frequent, with 60% of these experiencing at least some discomfort but only 10% categorizing their pain as severe. The incidence of the visceral type of pain was even less frequent. Overall, 20% reported pain in the severe range with a slightly higher percentage in those with paraplegia than in those with quadriplegia. In general, disabling pain has been more frequent in those with lumbosacral lesions (25).

In still another survey of hospitalized newly injured persons (26), the criteria for selection were those who received analgesic drugs on a regular basis or who frequently complained of pain. The quality of the pain was not defined. The percentage meeting these criteria varied between an SCI center in the United States and one in Australia. The much higher incidence in the United States was attributed at least in part to the greater use of laminectomy and posterior fusion. However, within the Australian group itself there was some variation, with a higher frequency in females and those of Southern European rather than British background. The existence of disability attributed to the presence of pain thus involves the person and his or her cultural characteristics as well as the type and degree of impairment.

What one calls pain involves the reaction of the person to the existence of an unpleasant sensation, usually associated with damage having occurred to oneself. The distinction is made between pain and the signal of tissue damage, which is called "nociception." In Sherrington's phrase, pain is the psychical adjunct of an imperative protective reflex (26). However, unlike acute pain, the character of chronic pain at or below the level of the spinal cord lesion is not a signal of tissue damage.

The importance of this distinction is illustrated by a case of a man with paraplegia at T4 with sensation absent below that level. Starting several weeks after his gunshot wound, he began to complain of shooting pain from the site of injury radiating down his legs and into the genital area. Pain was almost constant. When asked to describe his difficulties, he mentioned that the pain distracted him from getting things done and interfered with his ability to get around. However, what troubled him the most was that he was unclear as to what might be causing the pain. Before his injury pain meant to him that something was wrong and he should find out what it was in order to do something about it. He really wanted to know whether the pain he was experiencing was due to some underlying serious problem that he needed to do something about. Once reassured that the sensations were not the signal of something serious, he felt that he could live with it.

In any individual, the disabling aspect of pain and thus the goals of its treatment may vary. One person dealing with injury to the cauda equina with recurrent severe cramping pain was most concerned about the frequency of the episodes. Although the pain was extremely severe, it lasted for a very short time and occurred only during the day. His initial goal was to have at least 5 minutes of relief between the episodes. Only after having achieved a later goal of 20 minutes respite did he become concerned about the intensity of the pain. Another person with an incomplete cervical lesion had pain present intermittently throughout the day in both the fingers and the thighs. He had particular difficulty falling asleep at night. His goal was to be able to fall asleep within 60 minutes after having gone to bed without needing to use drugs or alcohol. Still another person with a lesion at T12 had both severe stabbing pain in the legs and burning pain in the buttocks. He found the burning pain particularly troublesome. He was able to function fairly well when the intensity of that pain remained at a level of 5/10. His goal was to have that lowered intensity of pain for the several hours necessary for him to transact personal business.

Once one determines the goals, one may then assess the appropriate means for achieving them. The unique character of pain is its susceptibility to modulation. Appropriate pharmacological treatment is determined to some degree, albeit not entirely, by the character of the impairment. In all instances, the particular medication, its dosage, and mode of administration will vary with the person in whom the problem occurs, although there are general principles by which particular classes of medications are selected.

Treatment of the radicular type pain is primarily based on the use of anticonvulsants. Carbamazepine has been particularly successful in relieving the lancinating quality of this pain. The usual dosage range is 600–1,200 mg in divided doses. Phenytoin, clonazepam, and valproate in appropriate subtoxic doses should be tried if carbamazepine is ineffective (27). Transcutaneous electrical neurostimulation (TENS) has been used to augment anticonvulsants in this group.

Mechanical pain may be expected to respond to nonsteroidal anti-inflammatory drugs. Trigger point injections and TENS are particularly helpful adjuncts, combined with exercises and other physical methods as in the case described later in this section.

The central pain syndrome is less susceptible to pharmacological treatment and requires a combination of methods. Tricyclic antidepressants are particularly helpful and presumably act by inhibiting the re-uptake of monamines (28). They thus augment the action of norepinephrine and serotonin. Serotonin acting at the dorsal horn of the spinal cord is the neurotransmitter within the endogenous pain modulating system (29). L-Tryptophan ingestion can elevate central serotonin levels, since the amino acid is a precursor.

Still another level of analysis is necessary to define the characteristics of an effective treatment program for the person with chronic pain. The element of "suffering" is the additional component. One cannot divorce the person experiencing the suffering related to the pain from either the definition of the disability or the process by which the problems are solved. The following cases illustrate the degree to which the individual can be crucial to the success of any regimen.

CASE REPORTS

G. F. is a 24-year-old man with a lesion at C6, with intact sensation to pinprick and touch. Burning pain present since early after the injury 4 years ago has become progressively more disabling. It was particularly severe on the anterolateral surface of both thighs and the fingers of both hands. It was worse at night and interfered with his sleep. He had been advised in the past to drink several beers at night but found that his alcohol consumption had been going up and had become less and less effective. He was concerned that he was drinking as many as four to six beers each night and several "rum and cokes" in order to sleep and had gained 25 pounds because of such consumption. His initial goal was to fall asleep at night within an hour without the use of alcohol and he was to keep a record of the times when he met his goals.

He reported having met his goal on five of the past 20 nights. Pain had apparently been less severe on those nights. Although it took longer than an hour for him to fall asleep, he was able nevertheless to avoid the use of alcohol on 17 nights. Only on three nights did he need to use as much alcohol as he had been using heretofore. What helped him to cut down his consumption was the record he was keeping. He began to realize, he said, that he may not have the pain every night. He began to hold off drinking unless he absolutely needed to. His goal remained the same: sleep 8 hours each night without needing more than an hour to fall asleep and to do so without the use of alcohol or other drugs.

Several months later, he reported that the pain in his legs was no longer a problem, although it continued to be present. He found that he could fall asleep despite it without using alcohol. He had discovered that it was helpful to lie on his right side and to bend his legs at the knees, which helped to prevent his legs from jumping and lessened the pain.

This case illustrates the value of having the person with the problem carry out the act of recording the times when his goals are being met. He began to change his perception of the degree of severity of his problem, and discovered alternatives to the use of drugs derived from his own experience. The impairments remain but the disabilities, in terms

CONTINUING CARE

of their interference with function, are minimized by virtue of participation of the person with the problem in defining goals, measuring times when they were met, and searching for the solutions.

J. M. is a 33-year-old man with a long-standing lesion at T5, with preservation of response to pinprick and temperature to T10. He had recent worsening of long-term pain in his back, starting at the level of his spinal fusion. Pain is almost always present, but it is intermittently more severe. These more severe episodes would start with a sharp, pinching sensation at the site of his fusion and then would shoot down to the tailbone. If this pain lasted as long as 60 seconds, it would then be followed by spasms of his abdominal muscles and lower extremities. The spasms interfered with his sitting in his wheelchair and would awaken him at night. He was unable to get out of the house because of these difficulties, despite the ingestion of 60 mg of diazepam each day in divided doses. His initial goal was to "feel well enough to go outdoors without taking any more diazepam than I already take."

One month later, he reported 3 days when he had met his goal. On those days, the pain did not last as long and therefore did not result in spasms. He noted that what may have helped on those days was a feeling of his back becoming looser after having heard a "popping" in it while carrying out his ordinary routine of stretching exercises. (These consisted of 10 repetitions with a 140-pound weight.) His goal for the next month was to increase the number of days on which he was able to go out while simultaneously reducing his diazepam to a total of 45 mg each day. He decided to continue the stretching exercises so as to achieve the "popping" sound and to do so several times each day.

At the end of the next month, he reported 8 days, several in a row, when he had done well enough to go out of the house. Pain was lasting as little as 15 seconds and therefore the spasms did not occur. He had added to his treatment ice rubs to numb the area in his back from which the pain seemed to arise when he would be awakened in the night. He continued to use the stretching exercises.

Over the next several months, the number of "good" days increased to as many as 19 each month, and he enrolled in a sports program as well. The pain is still something that happens. "I now have something to fall back on if the pain and the spasms get bad. I have worked out some stretching routines to break up the spasms so they don't get bad enough to interfere with what I want to do." He began to use the ice rub on a more regular basis when he would have pain at night after he had been sitting up all day. He modified his stretching exercises to do them with a smaller amount of weight, and would use them when he would first begin to feel pain during the day. He had been able to reduce the total dose of diazepam to 20 mg each day.

This case further illustrates the value of getting the person with the pain to participate in the process of managing it. This man was able to develop an entire repertoire of strategies for dealing with his problem. Although the procedures were not in themselves in any way unique, their application was effective because the person with the problem could fine-tune their use. The role of the professional in working with the person with chronic pain should be to encourage the development of the ability to manage oneself: to monitor one's own body and its reactions. Medication became far more effective as part of the total approach. When he was asked to evaluate the process of planning that had gone on, he felt that it had been particularly useful for him to be the one who had found out what worked for him. "I got a handle on myself. I was helped to keep in touch with myself."

REFERENCES

1. Ozer MN, Schmitt JK, eds (1987): *Medical Complications of Spinal Cord Injury*. Philadelphia: Hanley and Belfus. (Physical medicine and rehabilitation: state of the art reviews, vol 1, no. 3.)
2. Rossier A, Foo D, Shillito J, Dyro F (1985): Post-traumatic cervical syringomyelia. *Brain* 108:439–461.
3. Williams B, Terry A, Francis Jones H, McSweeny T (1981): Syringomyelia as a sequel to traumatic paraplegia. *Paraplagia* 19:67–80.
4. Dworkin G (1985): Post-traumatic syringomyelia. *Arch Phys Med Rehab* 66:329–331.
5. Gates P, Fox A, Barnett H (1986): CT metrizamide myelography in syringomyelia: sensitivity and specificity. *Neurology* 36:1245–1248.
6. Quencer R, Sheldon J, Post M, Diaz R, Mantalvo B, Green B, Eismont F (1986): Magnetic resonance imaging of the chronically injured cervical spinal cord. *Am J Neuroradiol* 7:457–464.
7. Stanworth P (1979): The significance of hyperhidrosis in patients with post-traumatic syringomyelia. *J Neurol Neurosurg Psychiatry* 42:962–963.
8. Watson N (1981): Ascending cystic degeneration of the cord after spinal cord injury. *Paraplegia* 19:89–95.
9. Dyro F, Rossier A (1983): Electrodiagnostic abnormalities in 15 patients with post-traumatic syringomyelia: pre- and postoperative studies. *Paraplegia* 23:233–242.
10. Lance JW (1980): Pathophysiology of spasticity and clinical experience with Baclofen. In: *Spasticity: Disordered Motor Control*, edited by Feldman RG, Young RR, Koella WP. Chicago: Year Book Medical Publishers, pp 185–203.

11. Dimitrijevic M, Nathan P (1967): Studies of spasticity in man: some features of spasticity. *Brain* 90:1–30.
12. Dimitrijevic M, Nathan P (1968): Studies of spasticity in man: 3. Analysis of reflex activity evoked by noxious cutaneous stimulation. *Brain* 91:349–368.
13. Dimitrijevic MR (1973): Withdrawal reflexes. In: *New Developments in Electromyography and Clinical Neurophysiology*, edited by Desmedt JE. Basel: Karger, pp 744–750.
14. Shahani BT, Young RF (1973): Human flexor spasms. In: *New Developments in EMG and Clinical Neurophysiology*, vol 3, edited by Desmedt J. Basel: Karger, pp 734–743.
15. Shahani B, Young R (1977): Further studies on flexor spasms. *EEG Clin Neurophysiol* 43:149.
16. Guttmann L (1952): Studies on the reflex activity of the isolated cord in spinal man. *J Nerv Ment Dis* 116:957.
17. Delwaide P (1985): Electrophysiological analysis of the mode of action of muscle relaxants in spasticity. *Ann Neurol* 17:90–95.
18. Davidoff R (1985): Antispasticity drugs: mechanisms of action. *Ann Neurol* 17:107–116.
19. Koella WP (1980): Baclofen: its general pharmacology and neuropharmacology. In: *Spasticity: Disordered Motor Control*, edited by Feldman RG, Young RR, Koella WP. Chicago: Year Book Medical Publishers, pp 383–396.
20. Kirkland L (1984): Baclofen dosage: a suggestion. *Arch Phys Med Rehab* 65:214.
21. Guttmann L (1973): *Spinal Cord Injuries: Comprehensive Management and Research*. London: Blackwell Scientific Publishers.
22. Cook AW, Nathan PW, Smith MC (1984): Sensory consequences of commissural myelotomy. *Brain* 107:547–568.
23. Donovan W, Dimitrijevic M, Dahm L, Dimitrijevic M (1982): Neurophysiological approaches to chronic pain following spinal cord injury. *Paraplegia* 20:135–146.
24. Woolsey RM (1986): Chronic pain following spinal cord injury. *J Am Paraplegia Soc* 9:39–41.
25. Nepomuceno C, Fine PR, Richards JS, et al. (1979): Pain in patients with spinal cord injury. *Arch Phys Med Rehab* 60:605–609.
26. Burke DC (1973): Pain in paraplegia. *Paraplegia* 10:297.
27. Farkash PE, Portenoy RK (1986): Pharmacological management of chronic pain in the paraplegic patient. *J Am Paraplegia Soc* 9:41–50.
28. Walsh TD (1983): Anti-depressants in chronic pain. *Clin Neuropharmacol* 6:271–288.
29. Hendler N (1982): The anatomy and psychopharmacology of chronic pain. *J Clin Psychiatry* 43:15–21.

CHAPTER 5

Participatory Planning

The approach to planning the collaborative management of problems in the rehabilitation and continuing care phases in the person with SCI complements the classic diagnostic approach used to manage acute care problems. The procedures useful in participatory planning are techniques that can be specified and learned, just as those for carrying out a physical examination were learned.

THE PROBLEM

It has been estimated that, if treatment is long-term and preventative in nature, instructions or recommendations are followed less than 50% of the time (1). This issue must be dealt with in terms of its effect on the outcomes of rehabilitation and health care. Failure to follow through with treatment programs may jeopardize the person's health, increase the costs of care by decreasing its efficiency, and interfere with research intended to determine treatment efficacy. The mode by which plans are generated is one aspect of the problem.

Follow-through is improved when a person's expectations regarding his treatment are met. This is more likely to occur when there is agreement between the patient's and the professional's expectations; involving the patient in goal setting increases follow-through (2). An individual is also more likely to see the relevance of the therapeutic program to his goals when statements are couched in functional terms. For example, it is helpful if the goal deals with "walking" rather than "increased strength in the quadriceps." Later measurement of the accomplishment of goals on the part of a patient is also more likely if they are stated in terms within that person's set of experiences. Participating in such evaluation helps one continue to generate the effort necessary for continued success (3).

Conversely, the patient's contribution to goal setting may lack the precision or specificity necessary for adequate delineation of either the problem or the goal; the professional's role is to aid the patient in making a more adequate statement of his goals. The more global the statement, the less likely the goal will be achieved given the relatively short-term nature of any rehabilitation program, and the less likely that there will be clear awareness of achievement if it does occur. For example, a global goal statement such as "walking" would be improved by being more "specific," such as "walking between parallel bars for 10 feet." Such a goal statement may be more short-term as well as more easily measured by both the patient and professional. The goal statement thus needs to be both functional and specific.

THE GOAL

The aim then is more effective collaboration in planning between the patient and the professional. The goals statement must arise from the patient to the maximal extent consistent with making these goals clear. Since the patient alone ultimately determines whether a goal is worth working for, the goals to be incorporated into the total plan must arise from the patient's needs. The goal statement must be made in terms the patient can understand and must be specific enough to be measured by both the patient and the professional. Further, the aim is for the patient to participate to the maximal degree in planning, and, by so doing, he will be more likely to take an equally active role in carrying out such plans and to expand his capabilities over time.

To meet the criterion of "specificity," the goal statement should contain as a minimum an answer to each of three questions: *what* outcome is to be achieved; *where* and *when* in terms of the setting in which it is to be achieved; and to *what degree* or *how much* in terms of some quantification. For example, a statement meeting this three-point criterion would be a goal such as "transfer from bed to chair within 10 minutes." This statement describes the action to be accomplished (transfer), the setting (from bed to chair), and to what degree (taking no more than 10 minutes). Another example would be a statement such as "maintain the intensity of pain below 5 on a scale of 0–10 during the night." This statement describes what is to be accomplished (maintain the intensity of pain), the setting (during the night), and to what degree (5/10).

Patient participation is determined by his opportunity to answer the questions posed. Table 5-1 describes the various levels of participation that can be achieved. "Maximal" patient participation is determined by starting at the highest level of choice and then going down the scale only one step at a time and doing so only as necessary in order to meet the

PARTICIPATORY PLANNING

TABLE 5-1. *Degrees of Patient Participation in Planning Process*

	Therapist	Patient	Percent contribution
Independence	—	Asks himself; answers for himself	100
Free choice	Asks open-ended questions without providing answers	Answers for himself; explores and selects	80
Multiple choice	Asks by providing several (three) answers; "suggests"	Selects answer(s) for himself	60
Forced choice	Asks by recommending (one) answer prior to action	Agrees (or disagrees) "yes" or "no"	40
No choice	Does not ask; prescribes; action predetermined	Compliant (or noncompliant)	20

criterion of specificity. In identifying the problem and the eventual goal, it is considered necessary to involve the patient on the level of "free choice" at the start. If this level of participation is not effective in achieving answers to the problem or goal statement, one may then move to the next lower level of participation signified by "multiple choice." Only if necessary would one move to the level of providing a single recommendation to which the patient is asked to agree (or disagree). It is undesirable and rarely ever necessary for the physician to function at the level of prescription in dealing with the definition of the problem and the goal statement during the rehabilitation and continuing care phases. Doing so gives the patient little role in planning, and thus there is little likelihood that the patient will participate in implementation. The procedure of starting at the top of the scale and going down one step at a time usually provides a greater degree of patient participation than one might have anticipated initially.

THE METHOD

The aim is to develop a plan for the management of an identified problem. This plan consists of a goal, a means for accomplishing that goal, and a time limit at the end of which the goals and the means will be evaluated and a new plan formulated for the future. Before determining goals, it is necessary to correctly identify the problem to be remedied.

TABLE 5-2. *Structure of the Planning Process*

EXPLORATION	1. What are your concerns?
	    a) Concern 1
	    b) Concern 2
	    c) Concern 3

SELECTION	2. What is your greatest concern?
	    a) What
	    b) Where or when
	    c) To what degree

EXPLORATION	3. What do you want to see happen? What would make you feel that you are making progress? What are your goals?
	    a) Goal 1
	    b) Goal 2
	    c) Goal 3

SELECTION	4. What is your specific goal?
	    a) What
	    b) Where or when
	    c) To what degree

This is the first step in involving the person who ultimately must be responsible for implementing the plan.

Planning can be more easily understood when the definitions of problem and goal are seen as a three-stage process: exploration, selection, and specification. The exploration stage includes generating a list of three answers with judgment suspended until one specifies the concern(s). The specified concern then provides the basis for developing the goal statement(s). Generating goal statement(s) should also explore several alternatives before selecting the one that has the highest priority or should be first. One may then specify that goal in accordance with the criteria established (*what, where or when, to what degree*). Table 5-2 delineates this planning format.

At the level of "free choice," the patient both generates the list and makes the selection from the list of options. At the level of "multiple choice," the patient makes the selection from a previously generated list. At the level of "forced choice," the patient merely agrees (or disagrees) to a selection already made.

The exploration stage should encourage a wider range of options than might ordinarily be done. Several problems may need to be incorporated into a number of plans. Initial exploration may also ensure that several concerns are considered before one or another is selected as having the highest priority. As an example, when a woman with left-sided weakness was asked about her problem, her first answer was "tingling on my left side." When asked for any other problems, she mentioned "trouble using my ankle." When asked once again, for the third time, she answered "I can't move my toes." When asked to select what bothers her the most, her statement was, "It's hard for me to walk," the statement that should be used as the basis for generating a possible goal.

Even more useful at times is the opportunity that exploration offers for transforming the discussion from impairments to focus on the functional consequences or disabilities. For example, when another woman with left-sided weakness was asked, "What is bothering you?", her answer was, "My left side is weak." When then asked, "What problems does the weakness on your left side cause you?", she replied, "I have trouble going up and down the steps." When asked for the third time: "What sort of trouble do you have in going up and down the steps?", she said, "I'm afraid I will lose my balance on my steep front steps." Once the functional problem has been explored, one may offer the various statements (generated in this instance in a "free choice" fashion) from which the patient can select her greatest concern or what she feels to be the best statment of her concern.

In delineating the problem in terms of the person's life, one is exploring it in depth just as one would with any chief complaint in medicine. The difference lies in the use of the data. The definition of the problem is used to generate an appropriate goal statement rather than to determine the anatomical locus of a problem. For example, in dealing with the issues of spasticity, one would explore with the patient not only the typology, duration, and the frequency of the complaint but also the activities with which it has interfered. The goal statement would include the criteria demonstrating alleviation of the problem.

The process of defining a problem is ongoing. The answers will, of course, vary with the individual's degree of impairment, type of impairment, and the individualistic setting in which he is required to function. The actual statement made by the patient may change over time as thoughts become clearer, as old problems are solved and new ones appear, and as he feels more trust in the person who is asking the question. The ability to answer this or any other question also depends on the skill of the person in verbalizing what he or she is thinking or feeling. The aim is to enable the patient to answer this question as freely as possible, recognizing the limited degree of success one may have in doing so at any one time.

It may be necessary to repeat the cycle of exploration and selection in order to define a problem worthy of creating a goal worth working toward. The short time generally available limits exploration at the start. Making exploration a threefold process has proved a useful compromise and an ongoing professional/patient relationship permits reopening this exploration whenever it appears indicated.

Once the problem has been identified to the satisfaction of the patient, one begins to explore possible goals. The first statement of goal is frequently quite global; and the goal may thus be also relatively long-term. Exploration at this point once again permits clarification of the goals including the identification of shorter-term goals more likely to be accomplished. The question can be phrased as: "What might be the first step in meeting your goal?" As an example, one patient stated her goal was to "walk on my own between the nurse's station and the therapy room." When asked to set an intermediate goal, she was at first unable to do so. When then offered several alternatives (multiple choice)—"walking while holding on to another person, using a walker, using a wheelchair to hold onto"—she was able to select one that suited her and the therapist.

Generally by the end of the first meeting between the professional and patient, the goal statement has been made clear and specific enough to be understood by both. The patient is encouraged to record the times the goal is met. For example, if the goal is to "control the spasms so that they don't interfere with my driving my chair during the day," the patient would record the days that goal is met.

During subsequent sessions, the degree to which the goals have been accomplished is reviewed. The generic question is, "What has been accomplished?" There may have been several days during the week when the goal was met. After three instances are described, the next question deals with the means by which the outcomes had been achieved. The generic question is, "What may have helped to bring about those results?" Focus on this question as potentially most productive in enlisting the patient in his own care. Until this point, focus has been on the patient contributing to the definition of his problem, his goals, and the measurement of their achievement. The patient for the first time has been asked to contribute to identifying the means by which those goals may be achieved (4).

After evaluating the degree of accomplishment and the means, there is an opportunity once again to explore new problems and to re-evaluate the goals. See Table 5-3 for the general structure of the planning/evaluation cycle.

The questions used in this planning approach differ from those traditionally used in medicine, since the patient is asked to participate in setting goals as well as defining problems. Once that has been done, one has the opportunity to ask the patient to participate in evaluating both

TABLE 5-3. *Structure of the Planning/Evaluation Cycle*

Initial planning
1. What are your concerns? What problems do you have?
    Explore concerns and problems
    Select the problem that bothers you the most or the aspect that is most troublesome to you
2. What would make you feel that you are making progress in dealing with your problem? What are some goals?
    When will we review?

Review session
1. What times have you met your goal?
2. What may have helped to bring about those results?
3. What problems are you now having?
    Explore problems
    Select the problem that bothers you the most or the aspect that is most some to you
4. What are some goals for the next interim?
    What means will you choose to achieve your goals?
    When will we review?

the effects of the therapy and the therapies themselves, which may have contributed to those effects. In the process of addressing these new questions, the patient can begin to see himself as an increasingly active partner with the professional in maintaining his health—the overall aim of the continuing care phase.

REFERENCES

1. DiMatteo MR, DiNicola DD (1982): *Achieving Patient Compliance.* New York: Pergamon Press.
2. Martin J, Tubbert P (1984): Behavioral management strategies for improving health and fitness. *J Cardiac Rehab* 4:200.
3. Payton O, Ivey J (1981): The role of psycho-education in allied health practice and education. *J Allied Health* 10:91–100.
4. Ozer M (1981): Planning with patients: a feedback loop engendering health. In: *Applied Systems and Cybernetics, Vol IV,* edited by Lasker GE. New York: Pergamon Press, p 1681.

Index

Abscess formation, spasticity as symptom, 93
Acute care, 6–8,10,13–26
   alignment, spinal, 19,20
   completeness of injury, 17,18
   CT scan, 19
   decompression, 19,20
   flow chart, 14
   goals, 13,22–26
   motor level classification, key muscles for, 15
   neurological aspects, 13–19
   orthopedic aspects of injury, 19–22
   sensory dermatomes for classification of level, 16
   spectrum of instability, 20–21
   zone of injury, 17–18
alpha-Adrenergic system
   agonists, 58
   blockers, 41,54,55,64
beta-Adrenergic system agonists, 58
Age and SCI, 5
Alcohol, 57,58
   chronic pain, 102
Alignment, spinal, acute care, 19,20
Ambulation, 67–69
   degree of, and rehabilitation, 34–35
Anal wink, 15,39,44,48
Anhidrosis, 52
Ankle–foot orthosis (AFO), 69
Anterior cord syndrome, 18,19
Anticonvulsants, 101
Antidepressants, tricyclic, 101
Anus
   patulous, 44
   wink reflex, 15,39,44,48
Areflexia, detrusor, 38,40,42
Arm supports, mobile, 74

Arterial blood supply, spinal cord, 5
Automatic reflex bladder, 57
Autonomic dysreflexia, 54–56
   bladder distension, 42,54,55
   rectal distension, 45,54,55,60
   sweating, 54,55
Autonomic hyperreflexia, 16
Autonomic nervous system
   diagram, 51
   function, and rehabilitation, 50–56

Baclofen, spasticity treatment, 95–97
Barthel Index, 78,79
Benzodiazepines, spasticity treatment, 95,96,103–104
Bethanacol sensitivity test, 42
Bladder
   automatic reflex, 57
   distension, autonomic dysreflexia, 42,54,55
   innervation and control, 17,24–25
   neurogenic, classification, 38
   retraining, 56–59
   spasticity management, 93
Blood–brain barrier, 95
Blood pressure, 50,53–55
Body temperature, 9,16,50,52–53
Bowel
   peristalsis paralysis, 25
   retraining, 59–60
   spasticity before movement, 94, 96
Braces, 67,69
Breasts, sexual stimulation, 63
Breathing, rehabilitation, 77–78
Brown-Sequard syndrome, 18,19
Bulbocavernosus reflex, 15,17,39,48

Caffeine, 57
Carbamazepine, chronic pain treatment, 101
Cardiovascular regulation, 50,53–54
Cars, 72
Case reports
 chronic pain management, 102–104
 post-traumatic syringomelia, 90–91
 spasticity management, 93–97
Catheter
 indwelling, 39,59
 intermittent, 57–59
Cauda equina syndrome, 17
Central cord syndrome, 18
Central pain, 99,101
Cervical halter, stretch test with traction, 21
Charcot-type joints, 89
Chronic pain management, 97–104
 case reports, 102–104
 goal setting, 100–102
Classification, SCI
 motor level, key muscles, 15
 sensory dermatomes and, 16
Clitoris, 47
Clonazepam, chronic pain treatment, 101
Completeness of injury, 13
 acute care, 17,18
Continuing care, 7,10,87–104
 chronic pain, 97–104
 health maximization as goal, 87
 impairment/disability relationship, 87
 self-management, 88,91
 spasticity management, 91–97
 syringomyelia, post-traumatic, 88–91
 See also Planning, participatory
Contraception, 47,49
 oral, contraindications, 47
Contractures, muscle, 25–26
 chronic pain management, 97
Counseling, sexual activity, 63
Crede maneuver, 57
Crutches, 67,69

CT scan, 19,89,90
Cutaneous stimuli, noxious, and spasticity management, 92
Cyst enlargement, 88–90

Daily living, rehabilitation, 73–77
Dantrolene, spasticity treatment, 95
Decompression, acute care, 19,20
Deep vein thrombosis, 22
Defecation, rehabilitation, 43–46
Detrusor
 areflexia, 38,40,42
  with sphincter disturbances, 42–43
 hyperreflexia, 38–40
Diaphragm, 77,78
Diazepam, spasticity treatment, 95, 96,103–104
Dietary fiber, 60–62
Disability/impairment, 4–5,9,87; *see also* Impairment
Dysreflexia, automonic, 54–56
 bladder distension, 42,54,55
 rectal distension, 45,54,55,60
 sweating, 54,55
Dyssynergia, 41–43,58

Electromyography (EMG), 40–43
Epidural hematoma, 20
Erections, penile, 17,47–50
 medical and surgical methods, 63–64
Exercises, stretching, 103

Fecal impaction, 43,44,59
Fertility, 49
Fiber, dietary, 60–62
Flexor spasms, spasticity management, 92
Follicle-stimulating hormone (FSH), 49–50
Footdrop, 68
Fractures, osteoporosis and, 9–10
Functional electrical stimulation, 67, 68,73,76

INDEX

GABA, 95
Gait cycle, 68–69
Guttmann's sign, 55

Halo-jacket, 21
Halo-vest, 20,23
Hand controller, 70
Hand function, 73–77
Handicap, 6
Harrington rods, 21
Heart rate, 50,54
Hematoma, epidural, 20
Heparin, 22
Heterotopic ossification, 22
Holdsworth theory, three-column modification, 21
Hydronephrosis, 40,41
Hyperhidrosis, 52
Hyperrflexia
   autonomic, 16
   detrusor, 38–40
Hypotension, orthostatic, 16,54
Hypothermia, 52
Hypoventilation, 77

Impairment/disability, 4–5,9
   continuing care, 87
   definitions, 30
   individual differences, 8–9
Incidence, SCI, 1
Independence, rehabilitation, 34
Individual differences, impairment, 8–9
Information-gathering, physician–patient interaction, 8–10
Ischemia, 64,65,67

Joints, Charcot-type, 89

Knee–ankle–foot orthosis (KAFO), 69
Kyphosis, 21

Laminectomy, 20
Ligamentous aspects of SCI, 19–22
Longitudinal level, SCI, 13,15,17
Lumbar root injury, 17
Luteinizing hormone (LH), 49–50

Magnetic resonance imaging (MRI), 89–91
Medical costs, SCI, 1
Men, sexual function, 46–50; *see also* Penis
Menstrual periods, 49
Micturition, rehabilitation, 37–43
   urodynamics, 39,40–43,59
Mobile arm supports, 74
Mobility retraining, 34,67–73
   safety, 67
Monoamines, 101
Motor changes, 89
Motor function impairment, rehabilitation, 32–37
Motor level classification, key muscles for, 15
Motor power, MRC scale, 35,36
Motor score index, 15
Mouth stick, 73–74
MRC scale, 35,36,75
Muscle(s)
   contracture, 25–26
   pain, 99
   quadriceps, 34–35,68
   shoulder, 36
   wrist, 37
Myelotomy, 98

Nasopharyngeal mucosa, stuffiness (Guttmann's sign), 55
Natural history, SCI, 6–7
Nerve conduction studies, 90
Neurogenic bladder, classification, 38
Neurological aspects, acute care, 13–19
Nociception, 100
Norepinephrine, 101

Occupational therapist, 73
Opiate antagonists, 22
Orthopedic aspects of SCI, acute care, 19–22
Orthosis, 23,67
   ankle–foot (AFO), 69
   knee–ankle–foot (KAFO), 69
   wrist–hand (WHO), 74–76

Orthostatic hypotension, 16,54
Osseous aspects of SCI, 19–22
Osteoporosis and fractures, 9–10

Pain
 chronic, 97–104
 four types of, 99–101
 muscular, 99
 post-traumatic syringomyelia, 89
Paraparesis/quadriparesis, 17
Paraplegia
 pressure sores, 64
 quadriplegia, 17
 survival rates, 3
Parasympathetic dysfunction, 17
Parturition, 55
Patient characteristics, SCI, 5–6; see also Planning, participatory
Penis
 ejaculation, 48,49
 erections, 17,47–50
  medical and surgical methods, 63–64
Peristalsis paralysis, bowel, 25
Personal care, 73
Phenoxybenzamine, 41
Phentolamine, 41,64
Phenytoin, chronic pain treatment, 101
Philadelphia collar, 23
Physician–patient interaction, information-gathering, 8–10; see also Planning, participatory
Pinprick response, chronic pain management, 98,102,103
Planning, participatory, 107–113
 follow-through with instructions, 107
 functional problems, identification, 110–112
 goal setting, 107–109,112
 patient participation, 108,109
 planning/evaluation cycle, 112, 113
 structure, 110
Posterior cord syndrome, 18,19
Posterior ligamentous complex disruption, 20

Prazosin, 41
Pressure sores, 25,64–67
Prevalence, SCI, 1
Priapism, 17
Proprioception, 89
Prostigmine, 49
Pulse, 50,54
PULSES profile, 78

Quadriceps muscle, 34–35,68
Quadriparesis/paraparesis, 17
Quadriplegia
 paraplegia, 17
 pressure sores, 64
 survival rates, 4
Quadriplegia Index of Function (QIF), 79

Radicular pain, 99,101
Range of motion, 15,26,35
Reconstructive hand surgery, 75–76
Rectum, distension and autonomic dysreflexia, 45,54,55,60
Reflex
 anal wink, 15,39,44,48
 bulbocavernosus, 15,17,39,48
 stretch, disinhibition, 91–92
Rehabilitation, 7,8,10,29–81
 autonomic function, 50–56
 bladder retraining, 56–59
 bowel retraining, 59–60
 defecation, 43–46
 breathing, 77–78
 daily living, 73–77
 education, 30,64
 goals, 78–81
  functional, by level of impairment, 33
 goal setting, 30
  individualized, 80–81
 impairments, defined, 30
 micturition, 37–43
  urodynamics, 39,40–43,59
 mobility retraining, 67–73
 motor function impairment, 32–37
  ambulation, degree of, 34–35
  classification, 37

INDEX

mobility, 34
scales, 78–81
sensation impairment, 31–32
sexual function, 46–50
sexual reintegration, 60,62–64
skin management, 64–67
thinking, reorganization of, 29–30

Safety, mobility retraining, 67
Scales, rehabilitation, 78–81
Scott-Craig brace, 69
Segmental, pain, 99,101
Self-management, 9,88,91
Sensation impairment, rehabilitation, 31–32
Sensorimotor/vasomotor disturbances, 15–16
Sensory dermatomes for classification of level, acute care, 16
Sepsis, 23
Serotonin, 101
Sertoli cells, 49
Sex and SCI, 5
Sexual activity/function, 17
  counseling, 63
  intercourse, 54
  men, 47–50
  rehabilitation, 46–50
    sexual reintegration, 60,62–64
  women, 47,63
Shock, spinal, 15,18,23–26,39
Shoulder
  muscles, 36
  range of motion, 26
Sitting
  difficulties in, post-traumatic syringomyelia, 89–90
  sores, 64
Skiing, 73
Skin management, rehabilitation, 64–67
Spasms
  flexor, spasticity management, 92
  post-traumatic syringomyelia, 90, 91
  treatment, and pain, 97
Spasticity management, continuing care, 91–97

Spectrum of instability, acute care, 20–21
Spinal alignment, 19,20
Spinal cord
  anatomy, 1–5
    cord segment-nerve root correlation, 2,3
  arterial blood supply, 5
  lamination of tracts, 4
  pain, 99,101
Spinal cord injury (SCI)
  age, 5
  common locations, 2
  complete/incomplete, 2,4
  incidence, 1
  longitudinal level, 13,15,17
  medical costs, 1
  natural history, 6–7
  patient characteristics, 5–6
  prevalence, 1
  sex, 5
  survival rates, 3–4
  transverse level (completeness), 13
Spinal shock, 15,18,23–26,39
Stretch reflex, disinhibition, 91–92
Stretch test with traction, cervical halter, 21
Stretching exercises, 103
Survival rates, SCI, 3–4
Sweat glands, 52
Sweating, 89
Sympathetic dysfunction, 15–16
Syringomyelia, post-traumatic, 88–91

Temperature, body (thermoregulation), 9,16,50,52–53
Tenodesis splints, 75
Tetraplegia, classification in, rehabilitation, 37
Thinking, reorganization of, rehabilitation, 29–30
Thrombosis
  deep vein, 22
  and OCs, 47
Tightness, spasticity, 93

Tongs in place with traction/halo-vest, cervical injuries, 20
Transcutaneous electrical neurostimulation (TENS), chronic pain treatment, 101
Transverse level of injury (completeness), 13
  and acute care, 17,18
Trapeze bar, 72,73
TRH, 22
Tricyclic antidepressants, chronic pain treatment, 101
L-Tryptophan, chronic pain treatment, 101

Valproate, chronic pain treatment, 101
Vans, 73
Vasomotor/sensorimotor disturbances, 15–16
Ventilator, mechanical, 77–78

Ventilatory impairment, 24
Visceral pain, 99,100

Wheelchair, 26,64,69–75,79,80
  backrest, 71
  interaction with environment, 69–71
  light-weight, 70
  modular, 70
  as prosthesis, 70
  seat, 70–72
  transferring to/from, 72
Women
  catheters, 59
  menstrual periods, 49
  sexual activity, 47,63
  sexual function, 46,49
Wrist–hand orthosis (WHO), 74–76
Wrist muscles, 37

Zone of injury, acute care, 17–18